025.066440

This book is due for return on or before the last date shown below.

Us
He

Using Web 2.0 for Health Information

edited by
Paula Younger and **Peter Morgan**

f facet publishing

Published by Facet Publishing,
7 Ridgmount Street, London WC1E 7AE
www.facetpublishing.co.uk

Facet Publishing is wholly owned by CILIP: the Chartered Institute of
Library and Information Professionals.

British Library Cataloguing in Publication Data
A catalogue record for this book is available
from the British Library.

ISBN 978-1-85604-731-9

First published 2011
Reprinted digitally thereafter

Text printed on FSC accredited material.

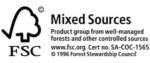

Mixed Sources
Product group from well-managed
forests and other controlled sources
www.fsc.org Cert no. SA-COC-1565
© 1996 Forest Stewardship Council
FSC

Typeset from editors' files by Facet Publishing Production in 10/13pt
Garamond and Frutiger.
Printed and made in Great Britain by MPG Books Group, UK.

Contents

Preface

The internet and the web have effected a profound and permanent change in our world and the way we view it. In both our professional and our social lives the consequences are with us every day as we try to evaluate, assimilate and utilize each new stage in the technological evolutionary process. Web 2.0 is the name used for convenience as a label for the present stage, in which the emphasis is increasingly on interactive communication and semantic enrichment. (Exactly what is meant by 'Web 2.0', and indeed whether such a concept as 'Web 2.0' really exists, is discussed in more detail in Chapter 2 'Web 2.0 in Healthcare Information: an overview'.) Web 2.0 applications are just beginning to reveal their potential as a way of improving and maintaining education and healthcare information in a wide range of situations, for caregivers and consumers alike.

Such is the pace of change, and such is the range of Web 2.0 tools and services on offer, that, while the journal literature provides an extensive coverage of recent developments, any attempt to produce a book surveying and summarizing the current state of affairs is inevitably destined to be overtaken by events. That certainty should not be seen as an argument against trying, though: the author or editor who waits for a more settled and stable state of affairs will in all probability be doomed to wait for ever. We share the belief of those others who have ventured into print in this area that there is a strong argument for providing the more considered, in-depth and reflective overview of web-based activities that a book makes possible; mapping key stages in the web's evolution, in the impact it has on our lives, and in the opportunities it enables us to grasp. Each book on the web is thus part of an incremental process of both advocacy and record. So, in formulating the case for this book we were – and remain – convinced that there is indeed a place for it and an audience that will benefit from reading it.

Let us first be clear as to what this book is not. It is not a manual designed to provide definitive and exhaustive instructions in how to develop or use Web 2.0 tools. The message throughout is suggestive rather than prescriptive. Instead, we have chosen to focus on a series of selective case studies, each written by contributors with practical experience and demonstrable expertise in their subject. Collectively they provide a synthesis of what Web 2.0 has to offer us in our professional (not to mention our social) lives. We have not attempted to cover every single aspect of the Web 2.0 world – there is no study of social tagging, or Facebook, for example – but many major applications are explored throughout the work, including wikis, blogs, RSS, podcasts and virtual learning environments. We intend that these studies should illustrate what is possible; explain how to assess whether a particular application is suitable for the reader's own situation; describe the sort of process that may typically be required in order to translate an idea into practice; evaluate and respond to the results; and, above all, hopefully inspire the reader to experiment and build on the work that our contributors and others like them have already carried out. While most of our professional work takes place in an essentially institutional setting, where service developments can all too easily be weakened, delayed or stifled by corporate policies and managerial procedures, one of the most stimulating characteristics of Web 2.0 tools is the manner in which they lend themselves to exploitation by individuals and informal teams possessing the enthusiasm, vision and ability to recognize the opportunity and seize the initiative. This democratization of effort can, of course, bring the strongly motivated individual into conflict with institutional practice, and so an important aspect of the case studies is the way in which they show how Web 2.0 applications can be harnessed and integrated into the institutional model.

While the case studies form the core of the book, they are preceded and followed by a series of contributions that provide a more reflective overview of the world of healthcare information, how it has embraced Web 2.0, and how it may evolve in future. These chapters establish the context in which we are working and provide a necessary framework for the specifics of the case studies. Here, too, we found it necessary to apply a degree of selectivity, notably in the area of Web 2.0 support for clinical care, where the most extensive applications have been developed by medical and other healthcare practitioners rather than from within the ranks of the healthcare information profession.

From the outset we were determined that the book should not be confined to a study of practice in the UK, our own home territory, but that it should have a strong international character. It would not be entirely correct to claim that the web knows no boundaries, since there are well publicized instances of countries attempting (whether for political, religious, cultural or economic reasons) to regulate or block the otherwise free flow of information across the internet. Nonetheless, in the healthcare information context it would be foolish to ignore the remarkable variety of web-based innovative practices found across different continents, and our international panel of contributors reflects that richness of variety. We should not forget, however, that different legislative frameworks apply in different countries, and that these may have a significant bearing, not only on the way in which Web 2.0 applications are administered locally, but also on the legal consequences of overstepping the permitted mark. Readers will need to recognize that this may in practice affect the way they can adopt and apply ideas from another country.

Contributors are drawn from a wide range of backgrounds: academic, public sector, research, and others. Approaches taken vary from the academic to the anecdotal, and environments range from large universities and research organizations to small publicly funded libraries. The chapters provide a snapshot of the state of Web 2.0 in the human healthcare information sector at the end of the first decade of the 21st century. As we move into the brave new world of 'Web Anywhere', these early days of what is sometimes currently termed 'Web 2.0' will come to seem as charmingly archaic as the early days of the internet seem to us now.

Our anticipated audience is large and varied. We feel confident that all healthcare information professionals – our primary target – will find something of value herein, whether they be senior managers or aspiring students, and whether they are already experienced in using Web 2.0 or novices exploring its possibilities for the first time. We also believe that a broader audience will find the book useful, since while the immediate focus is healthcare information, many of the case studies potentially have a more general relevance and could be adapted for use in other information environments. If the end result, for all our readers, is an improved understanding of the Web 2.0 world in which they work, we shall feel that this book has served a useful purpose.

Paula Younger
Peter Morgan

Acknowledgements

It is just over a year now that the idea for this book was proposed. I would like to thank my wife, Caroline, for her support over those months, and my long-suffering colleagues for their backing.

Peter Morgan

When I first encountered the internet in the mid 1990s, I had no idea how it would change my life: it just seemed like a fun place to 'hang out', an efficient medium for communication, and maybe to learn a few things. Now, I can't imagine a world without it. I certainly can't envisage how I could do my job efficiently if I didn't have access to the world's biggest library.

Just over a year ago, when I was asked if I would like to co-edit a book on the use of the internet in health information, I had no idea what a rollercoaster year lay ahead. I would like to thank Peter for his support throughout that time, and friends and family for putting up with somewhat curtailed visits and telephone calls over the last 12 months! I would also like to thank Facet Publishing for its support through the process: editing a book has proved to be a very different experience from writing the occasional article or review.

Paula Younger

Thanks must also go to all of our contributors for their willingness to participate, their punctuality, good humour and, above all, their help in creating this new publication.

Every effort has been made to contact the holders of any copyright material reproduced in this text, and thanks are due to them for permission to reproduce the material indicated. If there are any queries please contact the publisher.

Peter Morgan and Paula Younger

Contributors

Patricia Anderson

Patricia Anderson is the Emerging Technologies Librarian for the Health Sciences Library at the University of Michigan, Ann Arbor. In this role she advises users on effective and appropriate use of social media for enterprise purposes, as well as participating on and leading campus-wide social media teams. Her special interests include collaboration behaviours and supporting technologies, open science, web search behaviours and interfaces, web accessibility, plain language and health literacy, systematic review searching and evidence-based healthcare, and virtual worlds for healthcare support and education/research. She is the senior author of *The Medical Library Association Encyclopedic Guide to Searching and Finding Health Information on the Web*, and second author of the notable endodontics systematic review by Torabinejad (PMID: 17936128). In her earlier position as Head of the Dentistry Library she served as the systematic review searcher for 13 teams of the 2001 NIH Consensus Development Conference on Dental Caries. In October 2010, a team that she led received the Jean Sayre Innovation Award for the development of a plain language medical dictionary translation tool, made available as a Google Gadget and embeddable widget as a communication support tool for use by patients, clinicians and the general public.

Andrew Booth

Andrew Booth is Reader in Evidence Based Information Practice at the School of Health and Related Research (ScHARR), University of Sheffield. His research interests focus on all methods of evidence synthesis, evidence-based practice and knowledge translation. He has been involved in the development of a wide range of tools for dissemination, both web-based and as online briefings. He teaches on the University's Masters in Health Informatics and on the Masters in Public Health courses, specializing in Public Health Informatics and Use of Secondary Data Sources. He has a keen interest in e-learning and developed the Facilitated Online Learning Interactive Opportunity (FOLIO) programmes for the National Health Service and the Australian Library and Information Association (ALIA).

Andrew has authored over 120 peer-reviewed publications in a variety of health and information journals. He has co-edited three books: *Managing Knowledge in Health Services*, *Exploiting Knowledge in Health Services* and *Evidence-based Practice for Information Professionals: a handbook*. He is on the Editorial Team of *Health Information & Libraries Journal* and is also a member of the Editorial Boards of *Evidence Based Library and Information Practice*, *Journal of Electronic Resources in Medical Libraries* and *International Journal of Mixed Methods Approaches*.

He has worked in healthcare information for almost three decades in a variety of settings including the Medical Research Council, the National Health Service, the King's Fund Centre and now within an academic context.

Jon Brassey

Jon Brassey is Director of TRIP Database Ltd and ATTRACT, a clinical Q & A service, part of Public Health Wales (NHS). He has specialized for over ten years in the area of clinical knowledge management, with an emphasis on evidence-based practice. This interest started with the creation of the ATTRACT service in Gwent in 1997 – which sought to answer clinical questions based on the best available evidence. ATTRACT (www.attract.wales.nhs.uk) is still running and now serves all Wales. In addition Jon has been involved in numerous other Q & A services and his teams have answered over 10,000 clinical questions. However, Jon's most notable output has been the clinical search engine, the TRIP Database (www.tripdatabase.com) which has been searched over 50 million times since its creation in 1997-98. The main feature of his work has been to ensure that clinicians get the appropriate information to other clinicians with the minimum of effort and in a timely manner. Jon is currently working on a new project called TILT (Today I Learnt That), a shared learning project allowing clinicians to easily record and share their learning with other clinicians.

Sandy Campbell

Sandy Campbell is a Public Services Librarian at the University of Alberta John W. Scott Health Sciences Library, responsible for liaison to Medicine. Her professional interests include information consumerism and all forms of digital information services. Sandy has published and presented nationally and internationally on a variety of subjects, including information literacy and the collecting of electronic books and journals. She is a member of the Library Association of Alberta, the Canadian Library Association and the Polar Libraries Colloquy, and is an Associate Fellow of the Australian Library and Information Association.

Thane Chambers

Thane Chambers holds a joint appointment at the University of Alberta with the Faculty of Nursing and the John W. Scott Health Sciences Library as a Research

Librarian. Her research interests include instructional design and consumer health information behaviour. At work, she collaborates with and supports faculty members on research proposals and projects in the field of nursing. She has published on a range of topics, including designing instruction for Web 2.0 tools, using Web 2.0 tools in instruction, and exploring social media as an environment for teaching and learning.

Allan Cho

Allan Cho is a Program Services Librarian at the Irving K. Barber Learning Centre (IKBLC) within the University of British Columbia Library. His duties include the design and delivery of programmes and services to support academics as well as assisting in developing the IKBLC's online web resources, including integration of social media and virtual resources to support users. Allan read Chinese Canadian History for his Master of Arts degree and more recently completed a Master of Library and Information Sciences degree.

Allan has written articles on mashups, social cataloguing, Web 2.0 and Web 3.0. He is currently the editor of the Special Libraries Association (SLA) *Wired West* journal and authors Allan's Library blog (www.allanslibrary.com).

Laura Cobus-Kuo

Laura Cobus-Kuo has been Health Sciences Librarian at Ithaca College since August 2010. She previously held positions at the Health Professions Library at Hunter College in New York City and the Nursing Research Centre at the Jewish General Hospital in Montréal, Canada. She received her BA from the State University of New York at Albany, her MLIS from McGill University in Montréal, Canada, and her MPA from Baruch College of the City University of New York.

Laura presents and publishes on topics such as information literacy instruction, qualitative research, transdisciplinary research, evidence-based practice, curriculum design, web usability, Library 2.0 and Web 2.0. Her most recent journal contributions are in *Nursing Education Perspectives* on a transdisciplinary approach to integrating technology into a curriculum, *Medical Reference Service Quarterly* (MRSQ) on using blogs and wikis in public health instruction and *The Journal of the Medical Library Association* (JMLA) on information literacy instruction in public health.

Laura resides in Ithaca, NY with her husband and two-year old daughter and enjoys cooking, baking, jogging and yoga.

Pip Divall

Pip Divall is Clinical Librarian Service Manager at University Hospitals of Leicester NHS Trust. She is interested in mobile technologies, and has completed a systematic review of personal digital assistants in clinical care as part of her MSc in Health Services

Research at the University of Leicester (2010). Pip is also Conference Director for the Health Libraries Group branch of CILIP, and part of the organizing committee for the International Clinical Librarian Conference.

Jukka Englund

Jukka Englund has worked for over 30 years at the Terkko-Meilahti Campus Library (previously National Library of Health Sciences and Central Medical Library) of the Helsinki University Library, Finland. He is now head of information and IT services at the campus library. His and his team's work focus has been on making the electronic library as accessible and easy to use as possible for the user. The library has been offering internet-based services since 1989 and is currently concentrating on mobile and Web 2.0 services. Englund has published widely in Finnish medical and library science publications and has been in demand as a lecturer, both in Finland and internationally.

Dean Giustini

Dean Giustini is a health librarian at the UBC Biomedical Branch Library located at the Vancouver General Hospital. His duties include overall responsibility for the delivery of the hospital library's programmes and services, collection development, reference services and outreach. He has a Master of Education degree and a Master of Library Science degree.

Dean has written articles on teaching and learning, Web 2.0 and Web 3.0. He is currently the editor of the HLWIKI Canada (http://hlwiki.ca) and authors the *Open Medicine* blog and the *Search Principle* blog.

Chris Mavergames

Chris Mavergames is Web Operations Manager/Information Architect for The Cochrane Collaboration. Along with the Collaboration's Web Team, Chris manages the Collaboration's web presences, including cochrane.org and the platform that publishes more than 80 of the Collaboration's websites. Prior to joining Cochrane, Chris served as a metadata librarian at the British Library, working on the Archival Sound Recordings project (http://sounds.bl.uk), and as Director of Multimedia Services/Librarian at the New York City College of Technology.

Chris's background is in library and information science and he has an MLIS degree from Long Island University in New York. Chris contributed a chapter to a soon-to-be-released German e-health textbook on Web 2.0 and evidence-based medicine and has presented internationally on the topic of Web 2.0 and health information. He has extensive experience with Web 2.0 tools and technologies, with a research interest in the Semantic Web.

Peter Morgan

Peter Morgan is Head of Medical and Science Libraries, based in the Medical Library at Cambridge University Library, where he has spent most of his professional career following an MA in Librarianship at the University of Sheffield. He directed the project that established DSpace@Cambridge as the University's institutional repository, has led JISC-funded repository-based projects collaborating with chemistry researchers, and retains an active role in the areas of open access and repository policies. In the UK he was inaugural chairman of the University Medical School Librarians Group, has held office in other professional library organizations, and was Bishop and LeFanu Memorial Lecturer in 2000. He is currently a member of the UK Research Information Network's Consultative Group on Librarianship and Information Science, and is on the editorial board of the *New Review of Academic Librarianship*. He has been elected President of the European Association for Health Information and Libraries (EAHIL) for 2011–12, has worked for the British Council in Pakistan and Kuwait, and has presented papers at conferences across four continents. He has spent the past decade trying to keep pace with advances in web-based applications and to develop information services that capitalize on them.

Hannah Prince

Hannah Prince is Knowledge and Library Services Manager at the Princess Alexandra Hospital NHS Trust in Harlow, Essex, UK. She has worked in Harlow for nine years, after an MA in Librarianship at Sheffield University. As the manager of a small library, she is responsible for publicity, strategy and purchasing as well as literature searches, training and enquiry handling. She presented papers on e-journals at the CILIP Health Libraries Group conferences in 2008 and 2010. A member of local special interest groups on marketing, e-resources and library management systems, she particularly enjoys exploring new ideas and technologies, and finds Web 2.0 tools offer the most interesting opportunities for improving support for healthcare staff.

Dale Storie

Dale Storie is Public Services Librarian at the John W. Scott Health Sciences Library at the University of Alberta in Edmonton, Canada. As a liaison to the medical faculty and School of Public Health, he is regularly involved with systematic review searching and teaching evidence-based medicine. He has previously published or presented on blogging, gaming, information literacy and digital preservation, and is interested generally in the application of new technologies to library services and instruction. Although he makes frequent use of most Web 2.0 technologies on a personal and professional level, he still finds RSS to be one of his favourite tools, and is always glad to explore new ways of extending its usefulness.

Anthea Sutton

Anthea Sutton is an Information Specialist at the School of Health and Related Research (ScHARR), University of Sheffield. She is the programme manager for FOLIO (Facilitated Online Learning as an Interactive Opportunity) e-learning courses for information professionals, and has research interests in e-learning and literature searching. Anthea is also the Reviews Editor for *Health Information and Libraries Journal*.

Andy Tattersall

Andy Tattersall is an Information Specialist at the School of Health and Related Research (ScHARR), University of Sheffield. His areas of interest are using web tools and technologies to support research, collaboration and teaching. He is a keen advocate of Web 2.0 tools, cloud computing and the idea of using these platforms for informal and flexible working, learning and the propagation of creativity in education. Andy is also interested in the concept of visualization of data and recently reviewed David McCandless's *Information is Beautiful* book for CILIP's *MmIT Journal*. Andy has recently displayed a poster on 'Employing Web 2.0 Tools to Deliver E-learning Across Hemispheres' at the Future Learningscapes Conference in Greenwich. He has also presented at EAHIL (European Association for Health Information and Libraries) and Internet Librarian International on the topic of web portals such as Netvibes.

Paula Younger

Paula Younger is Library Manager at Weston Area Health Trust in North Somerset, the smallest NHS Acute Trust in the south-west of England. She was previously Electronic Resources Librarian at Exeter Health Library in Devon, after working for four years with the Ministry of Defence in the medical and science libraries in Hampshire and Wiltshire. Prior to that she worked for a training and enterprise council and a small electronic publishing company in the north-east of England before teaching English in Japan for two years. She is a qualified secondary school teacher and chartered librarian, with an MA in Information and Library Management from the University of Northumbria. She has a strong interest in new technology and its ability to make life easier and is always trying to persuade nurses and other clinical staff that the internet is really a useful tool.

Glossary

With thanks to Allan Cho and Dean Giustini for their contributions to the Glossary.

For a complete list of semantic search tools, see: http://hlwiki.slais.ubc.ca/index.php/Semantic_search.

ALIA Australian Library and Information Association.

augmented reality A live direct or indirect view of a real-world physical environment in which virtual, computer-generated imagery augments elements. The technology enhances the user's current perception of reality.

Blackboard A virtual learning environment used in many universities and other academic organizations around the world, allowing educators to make content available and manage classes online. Increasingly elements such as wikis, blogs, RSS and virtual-reality learning spaces are features of the system.

blog Short for 'weblog', blogs are one of the longest-established of the Web 2.0 technologies. A blog is an online journal, either literally an online diary or an account of activity in an organization. Most blogs are informal in tone. The majority are personal and/or non-commercial, although some companies and academic journals have launched their own blogs, for example the *New England Journal of Medicine* and the *BMJ* Group.

blogosphere Encompasses all blogs and their connections.

blogpost or blog post An entry in a blog.

BUPA British United Provident Association. Created in 1947, one of the UK's private health insurance companies.

CDC Centers for Disease Control and Prevention.

CILIP The Chartered Institute of Library and Information Professionals is the professional body for information professionals formed by the amalgamation of the Library Association and the Institute of Information Scientists in 2002.

CME Continuing medical education.

Cochrane Library Collection of databases and other data which synthesizes the results of reviews and research to make recommendations for interventions and treatments based on the best evidence.

Cognition Search (CS) CS uses natural language mapping and mathematical algorithms to locate content. Its technology helps computers to find meaning (or related concepts) and discerns relationships between words and phrases (meaning), paraphrases (a 'finger' or a 'digit') and taxonomies (a 'finger' is part of a 'hand', a 'cow' is a 'bovine' and a 'mammal'). CS searches across four domains: law, medicine, Wikipedia and the Bible.

COMPLIANT Contextual knowledge, Managerial skills, Professional skills, Learning and teaching, Interpersonal, and NHS (i.e. national health systems) context, and Technical skills. Competencies required by librarians and healthcare information professionals.

crowdsourcing The act of outsourcing tasks traditionally performed by employees or contractors to a group of people or a community.

Dublin Core (DC) (http://dublincore.org/) A metadata standard created by the Dublin Core Metadata Initiative (DCMI); it provides a semantic vocabulary for describing the 'core' properties of digital objects.

EAHIL European Association of Health Information and Libraries. This European organization aims to unite and motivate librarians and information officers to exchange best practice and knowledge.

Evri A semantic company changing how consumers discover content on the web. Some publishers using its semantic platform are the Washington Post, Hearst Publishing, Yahoo! and The Times of London. Evri has two million pages across 500 categories, content recommendation applications and a feature-rich API.

FOLIO Facilitated Online Learning as an Interactive Opportunity. A programme of online learning for health librarians.

folksonomy A system of classification derived from collaboratively assigning tags to categorize content on a website. Also sometimes referred to as social tagging.

Friend of a Friend (FOAF) An ontology language used to create machine-readable pages of metadata to describe people, the links between them and the things they create and do.

GIS Geographic Information Systems. In medicine, they may be used to track the location of an ambulance, for example.

haptics Referring to the sense of touch, haptic technology uses an operator's sense of touch to allow interaction via computer technology with virtual and remote objects. In medicine, haptic backs are examples of applications that have been used to allow learning by simulation.

hashtag Developed by Twitter users to make it easier to categorize Tweets. Prefixing a word with a hash symbol enables it to be used as a tag.

HINARI Health InterNetwork Access to Research Initiative. This is an initiative of the World Health Organisation (WHO) that focuses on the distribution of health information to developing countries. It provides free or highly subsidized access to major journals in biomedicine and related fields to non-profit organizations such as universities, hospitals, medical libraries and government offices in developing countries that meet eligibility criteria based on per capita Gross Domestic Product (GDP).

mashup A web page or application that combines elements from at least two different sources. Netvibes is an example of a Web 2.0 application that facilitates mashups.

metadata A set of descriptive elements about data (literally *data about data*) designed to facilitate resource discovery. There are three types of *metadata:* descriptive/content, structure/format and administrative/copyright.

microblog A broadcast medium in the form of a very short blog entry. Microblog entries can consist of short fragments of sentences, images or embedded video.

Netvibes A personalized, widget-based web publishing platform that uses a dashboard to provide integrated access to a set of digital resources.

NHS National Health Service. The NHS is the UK's national publicly funded healthcare service, established in 1948. The term also refers specifically to the service operating in England, while the equivalent services in the other parts of the UK – Scotland, Wales and Northern Ireland – have their own distinct variations of the name.

NHS Acute Trust An Acute Trust is the formally constituted body that manages a hospital in the NHS. The term may also be used to refer to the hospital in question.

NHS Evidence A web-based NHS service that provides all staff working in health and social care services with access to a range of health information supporting the delivery of quality patient care.

NHS Foundation Trust A Foundation Trust is an independent legal entity that manages an NHS hospital providing NHS care to NHS patients. As a self-governing organization it is free from central government control and able to determine its own future.

NHS Partnership Trust An NHS Trust that is responsible, often in collaboration with social services departments in local government authorities, for delivering mental health services.

NHS Trust A formally constituted NHS body responsible for managing an acute, primary care or mental health service.

ontology A description of characteristics of data elements and the relationships among them in a domain. Ontologies describe many more relationships between terms than thesauri, and multiple kinds of relationships among elements. Taxonomies tend to reveal hierarchical relationships only.

podcast A series of digital multimedia files that are delivered over the internet for playback on a computer or mobile device. Formerly known as a webcast, the name podcast reflects the subsequent popularity of the iPod for this purpose.

Powerset A semantic search tool applying natural language processing to search, aiming to unlock the meaning in ordinary human language. In the search box, express yourself in keywords, phrases or simple questions. On the results page, questions are answered directly and aggregated from multiple articles.

Primary Care Trust (PCT) The formally constituted body responsible for managing community-based, as opposed to hospital-based, NHS services.

PTSD Post-Traumatic Stress Disorder. A psychological disorder that results from exposure to a traumatic incident, such as may be experienced by military personnel in combat.

Pure Discovery A semantic search tool using the semantic tagline 'meaning matters'. It is a search engine that thinks and learns like us and interacts in a human way. Its KnowledgeGraph allows users to interact with a search tool conversationally, as opposed to using cryptic keywords.

Quatuo A semantic search tool that allows you to create, edit and publish your Friend of a Friend (FOAF) profile on the web. You can use Quatuo to search profiles and find relationships between people. By putting references on your FOAF profiles, you allow applications like Google to understand and reference your research.

Resource Description and Access (RDA) The new bibliographic description standard for libraries, archives, museums and information organizations. Built on the foundations of AACR2, RDA is a comprehensive set of guidelines for the description and access of print materials and digital media.

Resource Description Framework (RDF) A data model that allows relationships between data elements to be described in graph form and so that large-scale federation of data sources, taxonomies and ontologies is possible. It is also a model to define 'resources' (objects), the relationships between them and a semantic framework ('classification system'). RDF metadata is used in cataloguing to describe content and content relationships found on websites, web pages or in digital libraries.

RSS Really Simple Syndication (also known as Rich Site Summary). An automated web-based feed for distributing news and other updated information.

SDI Selective Dissemination of Information. A current awareness service, typically provided by a library, that provides clients with information on the latest publications in their specified area of interest.

Second Life A free, three-dimensional virtual world in which users, represented by avatars, can socialize, connect, and create and trade virtual property or services.

Semantic Protocol and RDF Query Language (SPARQL) The W3C's recommended standard for querying web data in RDF graphs. In RDF-based environments, graphical tools with SPARQL engines query hundreds of sources through a point-and-click interface.

Semantic Web A term coined by the W3C and Sir Tim Berners-Lee to describe a new stage in the evolution of the web in which data descriptions make it possible to federate, query, browse, and gather information from disparate internal and external sources. The result is a more complete and relevant set of data elements which are defined in statements called 'triplets', which contain a subject, predicate, and object.

semantics From the Greek to give signs, meaning, or to make significant. Semantics refers to aspects of meaning as expressed in language or other systems of signs.

SHA Strategic Health Authority. Currently the level of the NHS that sits between the Department of Health and local NHS Trusts. Due to be reorganized following the autumn 2010 UK Government Spending Review.

SHALL Strategic Health Authority Library Leads Group. A group of NHS librarians, each representing one of the Strategic Health Authorities providing strategic leadership to the NHS regions in England, that co-ordinates the management and development of library networks serving the NHS.

Truevert Truevert knows the meaning of words and how they are used. No taxonomies, ontologies, thesauri, dictionaries or author tagging are used. Searching takes minutes on a single computer rather than on a hundred CPUs. The tool is scalable and works in any language.

tweet A post on Twitter; limited to 140 characters and often sent from a mobile (cell) phone.

Twitter A website offering a worldwide social networking and microblogging service. Users can send messages ('tweets') via mobile (cell) phone or the internet.

Twitterverse The cyberspace universe occupied by Twitter and its users.

virtual reality An artificial but life-like environment created by computers and permitting interactive participation by the viewer.

virtual world A single instance of virtual reality that is defined by a specific set of characteristics.

Web 3.0 A contested term used by some to describe the third generation of the web from 2011 to 2020.

WHO World Health Organisation. Established in 1948, the WHO is the directing and co-ordinating authority for health within the United Nations system.

widget A small portable code element embedded in a web page that allows the user to customize or interact with a specific feature of the interface.

wiki A collaborative website that allows a group of users to share in creating, editing and commenting on content.

World Wide Web Consortium (W3C) Develops 'interoperable technologies (specifications, standards, software, and tools)' for enhancing the web including HTML, DHTML, XML and many others. See W3C's Semantic Web Health Care and Life Sciences (HCLS) Interest Group, http://esw.w3.org/HCLSIG.

WYSIWYG What You See Is What You Get. The term describes a computer–user interface in which what appears on the screen is broadly the same as the final output. It is commonly applied to word processing and desktop publishing applications.

XML eXtensible Mark-up Language. It defines a set of rules for marking up an electronic document in order to express semantic meanings in machine-readable form.

YouTube A website that allows users to upload, share, view and comment on videos. It is used predominantly by individuals, but institutions are increasingly employing it to distribute their own videos.

Introduction

Paula Younger

Since the internet first became widely available in the mid 1990s, it has established itself as the major source of information worldwide in many areas, including on some aspects of healthcare.

What has come to be occasionally termed, at least retrospectively, as Web 1.0 was the first incarnation of the internet. It was mainly text-based and very didactic, and subject experts were the only ones who made information available. A high level of technical skills was required to compose web pages, and access to the internet was only available from a limited number of wired connections and often very expensive.

The world in which we live now is very different. Anyone with a mobile device and a mobile internet connection can access the world wide web at any time. Content is more flexible and personalized, and no special skills are required to create a very effective wiki or blog, beyond a basic ability with ICT applications such as word processing.

Since it was first coined at the end of the 1990s, the term Web 2.0 has come, in certain circles, to provide a convenient umbrella term for a much more interactive and collaborative evolution of the internet.

In healthcare, Web 2.0 applications are just beginning to come into their own as a potential way to improve and maintain education and healthcare information in a wide range of situations, for caregivers and consumers alike. This book concentrates on the provision of healthcare to humans, and the theme of supporting clinical practice underpins many of the contributions.

The book is not intended as a manual, but rather as a snapshot overview of how some health organizations and professionals are using what are sometimes currently termed Web 2.0 applications and methods of working.

After an introductory overview to Web 2.0 and healthcare information, Part 2 of the book looks at some of the longer-range implications for the development of healthcare information. The investigations here incorporate case studies to illustrate the effective use and implementation of Web 2.0 applications. These range from wikis and blogs to RSS feeds and Twitter.

Part 3 includes case studies from a very practical point of view in a range of environments, and Part 4 aims to look into the future, where the Semantic Web, or Web 3.0, is already apparent as the next development of the internet.

Many major applications are explored throughout the book, including wikis, blogs, RSS, podcasts and virtual learning environments.

As a book about any aspects of technology tends to be out of date almost as soon as it is written, our authors have concentrated on the enduring lessons of their projects, particularly in the section of practical examples.

PART 1

The basics

CHAPTER 1

Health information: an overview

Peter Morgan and Paula Younger

What is health information?

Healthcare and medical information professionals have always been quick to adopt new technology (Kumar and Rawat, 2010; McKnight, 2005). This is, in part, due to the nature of their users: healthcare professionals require their information to be as up to date and accurate as possible. The consequences of not having such information to hand are laid out starkly by HIFA2015:

> Every day, tens of thousands of children, women and men die needlessly for want of simple, low-cost interventions – interventions that are often already locally available. A major contributing factor is that the mother, family caregiver or health worker does not have access to the information and knowledge they need, when they need it, to make appropriate decisions and save lives. (HIFA2015, c2010)

Lack of access to information remains a major barrier to knowledge-based healthcare in developing countries. The development of reliable, relevant, usable information can be represented as a system that requires co-operation among a wide range of professionals, including healthcare providers, policy makers, researchers, publishers, information professionals, indexers and systematic reviewers (Godlee et al., 2004).

Before we look in more detail at the potential for Web 2.0 to influence healthcare and medical information, it is pertinent to establish just what is meant by health information.

Broadly, health information consumers divide into two groups: those who deliver care, and those who receive it. Healthcare deliverers divide into two further broad groups: those who have direct contact with patients and those who make a difference to patient care indirectly. Medics, nurses and patient information professionals fall into the first group; librarians, managers, information professionals (including researchers) and health informatics professionals fall into the second group, in the majority of cases.

The direct deliverers subdivide into many further groups: qualified physicians and nurses, medical and nursing students, and allied health professionals are just some. Each group requires a different type of information: the qualified medics and nurses may require information to enable them to treat a patient, to enhance their own continuing professional development or to prepare a presentation, ward meeting, training session or board paper. Students, on the other hand, may simply require a brief overview of a condition or intervention in order to pass an assignment and build a foundation for their further career development. Members from each of these groups can be found in a wide range of locations: hospitals (or 'Trusts' as they are currently referred to in the UK); medical schools; family practice centres; community practices; research environments or private companies.

In terms of those who receive healthcare information, user categories include expert patients and those with no knowledge; and adults and children. All of these users have different information needs, depending upon their condition and other factors..

Web 2.0, with its flexibility, low cost, lack of need for specialized skills, and potential for collaboration and sharing, would seem to offer ideal opportunities to enhance the provision of information and education to healthcare deliverers and recipients alike. Before we go any further, however, it is helpful to place Web 2.0 in some kind of context. We therefore need to define healthcare information settings.

Healthcare information settings
UK NHS settings

The UK has had publicly funded healthcare via the National Health Service (NHS) since 1948. The NHS aims to ensure that consultations are free at the point of delivery, although patients often pay a contribution for their medications, depending on their level of income, and there is also the option to receive some treatments privately.

In the NHS, most healthcare information professionals work in a library located in an education centre: there are currently 389 NHS libraries listed in the Health Libraries and Information Services Directory (HLISD). NHS librarians will often work in close collaboration with the local universities that provide medical, nursing and other health-based education. A small number may also work collaboratively with universities in specialized research units; within patient information units; or in health informatics roles. A very small number work at Strategic Health Authority (SHA) level, offering advice in a regional context. Many health information professionals work in small special libraries within hospitals or other secondary care establishments, providing books and other information to staff, students on placement and, occasionally, members of the public.

Their roles vary, from the traditional librarian/library manager to the clinical librarian. Some libraries employ specialist trainers or electronic resources librarians. Typically, an NHS librarian will perform some traditional work, such as cataloguing and classification, but the majority of their work will involve collating information via literature searches and current awareness; and user education, whether that takes the form of inductions or dedicated sessions. Staffing levels are generally quite low, ranging from two or three employees in smaller organizations with up to 2000 users, to larger staff teams in libraries at the bigger teaching hospitals, such as University Hospitals Leicester, where they reflect the larger user base of over 12,000 staff. Healthcare staff may be physicians, nurses, allied health professionals (including physiotherapists and dentists), and student users will be training to enter those professions.

Many NHS library services also serve the local Primary Care Trusts, and in some cases the General (Family) Practitioner (GP) groups, although in practice GPs do not make much use of library services (Cullen, 2002).

This range of information profession roles is reflected in other countries, where they include clinical or hospital librarians, consumer health librarians, and more traditional roles such as cataloguers or circulation librarians.

Other healthcare information settings

A small number of health information professionals also work within research teams and in other settings, including in places other than hospitals and doctors' surgeries. Such settings include the uniformed armed services, government science laboratories, commercial companies and health insurance organizations.

Health information for patients/healthcare consumers

In the majority of cases, medical librarians do not come into direct contact with members of the public. It can therefore occasionally be difficult to remember that we are, ultimately, there to improve patient care. Our main task is to ensure that medical professionals have access to timely and accurate information to support their practice. Since the early 2000s in particular there have been examples of public and NHS libraries working together (Nair, 2006). The role of Web 2.0 in patient information and public health is explored in more detail in Chapter 7.

The role of information professionals

Information professionals must aim to ensure that healthcare professionals are able to access information compiled by people with sufficient knowledge to make the data authoritative. We must also ensure that users have the critical appraisal tools to decide whether the information provided is of high enough quality for use in treating patients.

We must not lose sight of the fact that the ultimate aim is always the most effective treatments/interventions for patients. In James Gunn's novel *The Immortals* (1962) there is a description of how computers might revolutionize medicine: an intern carries his entire medical library in his ambulance and depends upon it for diagnosis and treatment. Although this scenario is still rather remote, many providers, including PubMed and UpToDate, offer PDA versions of their applications. Web 2.0, combined with the iPad, Twitter and all that will come after, would seem to be a huge step towards this very responsive and personalized mode of providing healthcare.

We are now witnessing an entire generation who have never known a world without the internet. For the Net or iPod Generation, Generation Y, or the Millennials, the internet has been the main source of their information for educational purposes (Weiler, 2005).

Concern has been expressed by some medical professionals about the quality of health information on the internet in general (Scullard, Peacock and Davies, 2010) and on Web 2.0 sites in particular (Lacovara, 2008). Some other schools of thought, however, regard the best of the Web 2.0 sites as a valid source of health information (Laurent and Vickers, 2009). Still others concede that there is some useful information to be found in Wikipedia, but that dedicated medical information databases are better (Leithner et al., 2010)

There are a range of situations where Web 2.0 applications can be, and are being, incorporated into the delivery of healthcare information. These include outreach, education, promotion, engaging with users, information literacy, knowledge management, journal clubs, patient and consumer support, online collaboration, provision of tables of contents and other selective dissemination of information. In Part 3 of the book, projects in some of these environments are examined in more detail, through practical, real-world examples and case studies.

References and further reading

Cullen, R. J. (2002) In Search of Evidence: family practitioners' use of the internet for clinical information, *Journal of the Medical Library Association*, **90** (4), 370–9.

Godlee, F. et al. (2004) Can We Achieve Health Information for All by 2015?, *The Lancet*, **364** (9430), 295–300.

Gunn, J. (1962) *The Immortals*, Bantam.

HIFA2015 (c.2010) A Global Campaign: Healthcare Information for All by 2015, www.hifa2015.org/about/why-hifa2015-is-needed.

Hill, P. (2008) *Report of a National Review of NHS Library Services in England: from knowledge to health in the 21st Century*, National Library for Health, www.library.nhs.uk/aboutnlh/review.

Kumar, P. M. and Rawat, P. P. (2010) *A Proposal for Clinical Librarians in the Era of Evidence Based Healthcare, a need but a neglected profession: an experience*, http://espace.uq.edu.au/eserv/UQ:179871/n5_6_Thurs_Kumar_227.pdf.

Lacovara, J. E. (2008) When Searching for the Evidence, Stop Using Wikipedia! *Medsurg Nursing: The Journal of Adult Health.*, **17** (3), 153.

Laurent, M. R. and Vickers, T. J. (2009) Seeking Health Information Online: does Wikipedia matter? *Journal of the American Medical Informatics Association*, **16** (4), 471–9.

Leithner, A., Maurer-Ertl, W., Glehr, M., Friesenbichler, J., Leithner, K. and Windhager, R. (2010) Wikipedia and Osteosarcoma: a trustworthy patients' information? *Journal of the American Medical Informatics Association*, **17** (4), 373–4.

McKnight, M. (2005) Librarians, Informaticists, Informationists, and Other Information Professionals in Biomedicine and the Health Sciences: what do they do?, *Journal of Hospital Librarianship*, **5** (1), 13–29.

Nair, R. (2006) Access to Health: an NHS/public libraries partnership, *Library and Information Update*, **5** (5), 25.

Scullard, P., Peacock, C. and Davies, P. (2010) Googling Children's Health: reliability of medical advice on the internet, *Archives of Disease in Childhood*, **95** (8), 580–2.

Weiler, A. (2005) Information-seeking Behavior in Generation Y Students: motivation, critical thinking, and learning theory, *Journal of Academic Librarianship*, **31** (1), 46–53.

CHAPTER 2

Web 2.0 in healthcare information: an overview

Paula Younger

In the beginning . . . a brief history of the internet

Although the internet as we know it is relatively young, having existed in its current form since about 1995, the concept of a connected network of information and linked ideas has been around for at least 60 years (Bush, 1945). Physicians were highlighted, in particular, as a group who would find the 'memex' extremely useful. During the 1960s to the 1980s, what we now know as the world wide web continued to develop, incorporating e-mail and early webcams and, more recently, the participatory software and virtual environments that form the backbone of what can be termed 'Web 2.0'.

In 1990, Tim Berners-Lee and CERN implemented a hypertext system with the aim of providing efficient and timely information to the research community. Two implicit aims of the internet, linking community and improving the availability of information, were apparent in the system's creation.

Since it first took form in the early 1960s, the internet has evolved at an exponential rate. In 1994 there were just over 20 million users worldwide; by 2009 there were over 1.5 billion (World Bank, 2010). In the mid 1990s, what we now know as the world wide web first took form, and it has since become the information tool of choice for many. In the process, the internet has changed society and the ways in which we interact beyond all recognition (Naughton, 2006).

The mid 1990s were a clear turning point. What had been a specialized, text-based information environment became transformed into a more accessible and interactive platform. The first sale on Echo Bay's Auction Bay, precursor of eBay, occurred in 1994 (Collins, 2010). Crucially, 1996 saw the first web-based free e-mail service, Hotmail (Sharma, 2009), changing the way in which we communicate for ever. In 1994, graphical web browsers as a whole, which make the internet as we now know it so accessible and interactive, were still in their infancy: the current search engine favourite, Google, was still four years away (Boulton, 2009). Now that we live in a world of potential constant connectivity and mobile multimedia 'on demand', the early years of the internet seem charmingly primitive.

Web 1.0 to Web 2.0

Traditionally, new releases of computer software have featured version numbering along the lines of 1.0, 2.0, 2.2 and so on, and the phrase 'Web 2.0' references this. Some work sectors have adopted the 2.0 suffix: Classroom 2.0, Enterprise 2.0, Health 2.0 and Library 2.0 have all entered the English language (Boxen, 2008). Although the term 'Web 1.0' is occasionally used, it is debatable whether Web 1.0 actually ever existed, or whether the term is simply a retrospective one, used, for the sake of convenience, to refer to applications from the early days of the internet.

For some, Web 2.0 is just jargon (Hinchcliffe, 2006). For those who believe differences can be identified, Web 1.0 is much more didactic and offers less of a user experience than Web 2.0 (O'Reilly, 2005). In the O'Reilly view, Encyclopaedia Britannica was a Web 1.0 application. Experts provided information which was then sold to users. In the Web 2.0 world, Wikipedia is the new model, relying heavily on volunteer authors and editors, with a small editorial panel who moderate any obviously incorrect or contentious entries. In the Web 1.0 pattern, users set up personal websites on platforms such as Geocities (now defunct) (Wikipedia, 2009). In the Web 2.0 world, blogging offers a fuller experience than a simple web page. Viewers can leave comments and interact with authors. Social networking sites such as MySpace and Facebook offer further networking opportunities.

Other differences include wired (Web 1.0) versus wireless (Web 2.0); companies versus communities; owning versus sharing; and hardware costs versus bandwidth (Dittems, 2008).

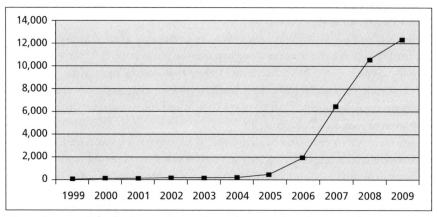

Figure 2.1 *Number of references to 'Web 2.0' from Google Scholar, 1999 to 2009*

Over the last ten years the number of scholarly articles written about Web 2.0 has increased dramatically, as the graph in Figure 2.1 shows.

The 2.0 phenomenon

Web 2.0 is not the only term that is now bandied about by journalists and others in an attempt to name and define the phenomenon of the next step forward in internet applications and modes of use. Other terms that have come into general use include:

- Health 2.0
- Library 2.0
- Medicine 2.0.

Although it is beyond the scope of this work to examine these in depth, it is pertinent to outline each one briefly.

Health 2.0

Wikipedia offers a 'concise definition of Health 2.0' as 'the use of a specific set of Web tools (blogs, Podcasts, tagging, search, wikis, etc) by actors in health care including doctors, patients, and scientists, using principles of open source and generation of content by users, and the power of networks in order to personalize health care, collaborate, and promote health education' (Wikipedia, 2010, citing Hughes et al., 2008).

Some authors describe five major themes of Health 2.0: participants are health givers and patients; it has an impact on both traditional and collaborative practices; it has the potential to provide personalized healthcare; it can also promote ongoing education in medicine; and as a less positive theme, there is possibility potential for inaccuracy in content generated by the end-user (Hughes et al., 2008).

Medicine 2.0

As A concept, some authors use the same definitions for Medicine 2.0 as for Health 2.0. It still refers to actors in health care, including doctors, patients, and scientists, using principles of open source and generation of content by users, and the power of networks in order to personalize health care, collaborate, and promote health education (Hughes et al., 2008). Other authors take an even broader view, regarding it as the latest tool and approach to ensure a better health system and well-being of humanity as a whole: 'health for all, and a healthy community' (Gavgani and Mohan, 2008). Eysenbach (2008) outlines five components that make up Medicine 2.0, which are defined as social networking, collaboration, participation, apomediation, and openness. Social networking, which includes the use of websites such as Facebook and LinkedIn, allows health professionals to interact with colleagues and peers and, potentially, with patients. The first approach is to use intermediaries, such as health professionals, to find relevant information to give to users, for example to patients. The second option is to use unmediated information that has not necessarily been validated in any way. Collaboration, participation and openness are self-explanatory;

Eysenbach describes 'apomediation' as characterizing the third way in which users can access credible health information, on the web.

Library 2.0

The term Library 2.0 was coined by Michael Casey, appropriately, on his LibraryCrunch blog (Chad and Miller, 2005). Chad and Miller again highlight the key features of Library 2.0 as being interactive, collaborative, and incorporating the use of multimedia web-based technologies. The focus on the user in this 2.0 world is very apparent (Casey and Savastinuk, 2007).

Whether it is Health, Library or Medicine 2.0, the phenomenon:

- is user centric: users contribute to the creation of the content and services they view
- incorporates multimedia; it is not just static text
- involves the use of networks and interaction with others
- involves personalized content
- requires care to be exercised in evaluating the content.

Specific applications often mentioned in the context of Web 2.0, Library 2.0 and Medicine 2.0 include blogs, wikis, social bookmarking, folksonomies and RSS, all of which facilitate the exchange of information and sharing of knowledge.

Web 2.0

The umbrella term Web 2.0 incorporates all of the above terms and more. The term entered common parlance after the first O'Reilly Media Web 2.0 conference in 2004 (O'Reilly, 2005). Above all, Web 2.0 is about collaboration, co-operation and sharing. At the institutional level, it is necessary to identify what to share, how to share, when to share and with whom to share (Kent, 2008).

There are far too many Web 2.0 applications to list or outline in any great depth, but this chapter outlines some of the ways in which health libraries and information professionals around the world are utilizing some of the most common ones to develop and enhance their services.

Librarians have always innovated and moved to adapt to new technology so as to provide more responsive services to their users: Web 2.0 simply represents the latest stage in that continuum.

What is Web 2.0?

In 2009, 'Web 2.0' became the 1,000,000th official term in the English language (MacIntyre, 2009). It was originally coined in 1999 (DiNucci, 1999) and the first attempt to define it was in 2004, when O'Reilly Media and MediaLive hosted the first Web 2.0 conference. John Battelle and Tim O'Reilly described their vision of the 'Web as platform' (O'Reilly and Battelle, 2009). Content became more collaborative; software applications were built that took advantage of internet connectivity, in a move away from applications and data on the desktop. Crucially, these new applications were easy to use: little, if any, programming skill was required. Anyone with good basic ICT literacy could now create web content, including blog posts, wiki entries, social bookmarking sites, or mashups.

Web 2.0 remains, however, obstinately difficult to define. Some definitions include 'the collaborative web' (Kamel Boulos, Maramba and Wheeler, 2006) and the 'read-write web' (Richardson, 2005–6). Some refer to a 'collection of approaches': new approaches to old problems (Spool, 2007). Perhaps one of the best and simplest descriptions of Web 2.0 is that it is 'all about harnessing collective intelligence' (O'Reilly and Battelle, 2009), a concept explored in more depth by Surowiecki (Surowiecki, 2004).

Many information professionals recognize the term Web 2.0, even if they are unsure what it encompasses. For many academics and health professionals, using terms for the individual applications, such as wiki or blog, may be clearer. A PubMed search for 'blog', for example, gives 171 hits; 'wiki' gives 111; 'Web 2.0' gives just 164, of which 8 include the term 'wiki' and 11 include the word 'blog' (search, 13 June 2010).

In some areas of medicine and healthcare, Web 2.0 is beginning to emerge as a mechanism for sharing information and working collaboratively – replicating online the way in which many healthcare and medical professionals interact in the physical world (Giustini, 2006).

This concept of the world wide web as a place where information and experience are shared represents a shift from the early days of the internet, where the creator (often described as the 'webmaster' or 'webmistress') was very much in charge (Guy, 2006). Most internet users still do not contribute online content: the 1% rule suggests that for every 100 people using online resources, 1 will create content, 10 will 'interact', and the other 89 will simply view (Arthur, 2006).

For the purposes of this collection, 'Web 2.0' is used as a convenient umbrella term to refer to a range of applications and ways of working. They are characterized by their potential for collaboration, whether in real time or in an asynchronous manner, and by their ease of use; no special technical skills are required to use them. Another key characteristic is that applications can be accessed from any internet-enabled machine: users are no longer tied to one particular place.

Web 2.0 is sometimes referred to by other names, including the participatory web and the read-write web. Future developments, already apparent, will include the semantic web, the mobile web and what might be termed the ubiquitous web ('web everywhere').

The keys to the future: some commonly used Web 2.0 applications

Anderson (2007) has outlined some of the most commonly used and key Web 2.0 applications, which include:

- blogs
- file and image sharing applications
- microblogging
- podcasting and vodcasting
- RSS
- social bookmarking, citation sharing and folksonomies
- social networking sites
- virtual worlds
- wikis
- really miscellaneous.

In this chapter, the ways in which healthcare information professionals are currently using some of these applications and modes of working are briefly outlined.

Around the world in 80 blogs: an international overview of Web 2.0 in healthcare information settings

As ever, the USA leads the field on Web 2.0. The Medical Library Association's website incorporates webcasts and an online boot camp for new health sciences librarians. Many American libraries have a presence on Facebook, including Weill Cornell Medical College and Yale University. Some institutions use Facebook to advertise training sessions and opening hours and to incorporate video inductions into their pages. Other libraries make use of Twitter: the TCMC Medical Library, for example, has used the medium to advertise details of clinical trials recently added to databases, book signings and subject guides.

The UK is, however, not far behind. Some extremely innovative work with Web 2.0 tools has been done at some of the larger teaching hospitals, notably University Hospital Leicester, which have implemented blogs, Twitter and an online journal club and taken part in cross-continental podcasts to encourage other clinical librarians. Shrewsbury and Telford Hospital Trust has also established a blog and an excellent mashup site, making very creative use of Netvibes. The FADE Library in Liverpool also has a long-established grey literature blog, and the Newham University Hospital NHS Trust also has its own blog. In Wales, Powys Teaching Health Board has set up an online journal club making use of a wiki. Increasingly, UK libraries have a presence on Facebook, although they are mainly those that have a strong university connection, such as the Rockefeller Library, or independent organizations, such as the Manchester Medical School.

In Europe too, rapid progress has been made, with Web 2.0 tools increasingly being adopted by a wide range of organizations. Webicinia has made it possible to deliver RSS feeds in languages that are not limited to English, for example ScienceRoll in Sweden (http://scienceroll.com/2010/09/28/swedish-collection-of-medical-social-media-resources/). The French health website Santelog incorporates podcasts and RSS feeds.

In the southern hemisphere, Web 2.0 tools have come into their own in the arena of delivering health librarianship and information services over vast distances. In Australia, blogs have been used to reach users in isolated areas (Keast, 2009).

In the developing world, access to the robust communications infrastructure required for the effective provision of healthcare information remains problematic (Wootton, Patil and Ho, 2009). With the advent of HIFA2015 (Healthcare Information for All, 2009), several projects have taken place in South America, Africa and other developing areas. There is also increasing awareness of the potential of social media and mobile technology to address this gap in coverage, although little published research is as yet available (McNab, 2009).

Guerrilla websites: the use of wikis as websites, intranets and repositories of information

Ward Cunningham, who created the original wiki in 1994, originally described a wiki as 'the simplest online database that could possibly work'. Other definitions describe a set of web pages easily edited by anyone allowed access (Ebersbach et al., 2006). Information on a wiki may be available to the world, as with Wikipedia, or limited only to invited guests, as is the case with some health and medical wikis. Equally, for some wikis, anyone can register and edit content, whereas only those with appropriate credentials may register and change entries on others.

There are sports wikis and how-to wikis, music score wikis and dress pattern wikis, and even a wiki about Harry Potter. The most famous wiki is undoubtedly Wikipedia, launched in January 2001 by Jimbo Wales and Larry Sanger. This collaborative encyclopedia has rapidly become one of the most popular reference sources on the internet. Academic views on Wikipedia are mixed, with some users finding it a valid source of information (Giles, 2005) and others finding it more contentious (Pho, 2009).

In healthcare, wikis can be and have been used to set up collaborative classroom projects and 'wikibooks', and as content management systems for policy documents. They have also been used to run virtual online journal clubs (Lizarondo et al., 2010) and to provide a world-class commissioning wiki, incorporating an information base compiled by health information professionals to support national health policy (Bryant et al., 2009). They have been used to facilitate group projects in nursing education and could be used to facilitate writing assignments and committee work (Billings, 2009; Kardong-Edgren et al., 2009). In addition to teaching practical IT skills in a cost-effective and real-time environment, wikis also enable learners to gain and practise skills required for working in a group (Ciesielka, 2008). Like blogs, wikis have also been used on occasion to explore the potential of providing a website for library patrons and healthcare information seekers (Hilska-Keinänen, 2009; Kraft, 2010).

Some particularly good examples of how wikis can be used in healthcare are the ECGpedia at http://en.ecgpedia.org/wiki/Main_Page and Human Physiology at http://en.wikibooks.org/wiki/Human_Physiology. Wikis are, however, not spread across all areas evenly: they are not common, for example, in mental health (Bastida et al., 2010).

There are other specific nursing and medical wikis, including the Rogerian nursing science wiki website, at http://rogeriannursingscience.wikispaces.com/, AskDr Wiki and ganfyd. A detailed list of over 65 medical and health wikis is available at the website of medical librarian David Rothman (Rothman, 2009).

Wikis have many advantages. They require no special skills to edit; users can access them from any internet-enabled device; users do not need to worry about backing up data, or about spam; and, as with the majority of Web 2.0 applications, they are designed to integrate other technologies, such as RSS. In addition, basic versions are usually free.

The portable online filing cabinet

Further uses of wikis in healthcare information environments include management of documentation required to keep a department running 24/7 (Meenan et al., 2010), the establishment of a faculty publications database (Connor, 2008), and support for an online health management course outlining how to document procedures effectively (Harris and Zeng, 2008). Again, the overall theme is collaboration, together with the ease of use of wiki software in general. Where providers of healthcare information need to work across more than one organization with more than one network, wikis can offer a very cost-effective method of circumventing IT barriers. The Library and Information Science Wiki (LIS Wiki) provides an extensive list of medical, healthcare and medical librarianship wikis, illustrating the range of wikis available and their myriad uses (http://liswiki.org/wiki/Weblogs_-_Medical_Librarianship).

Extending the reach of the service: Web 2.0 in outreach work

Reaching non-users, or those unable to physically make it to the library, has always been somewhat difficult. Web 2.0 makes it slightly easier to do this. As has already been mentioned, in Australia blogs have made it possible to reach people in rural areas. In the USA, Operation Medical Libraries uses a blog (http://operationmedicallibraries. blogspot.com/) and a Facebook page to facilitate the provision of medical information to those in the military in remote areas; and in singleton services Web 2.0 makes it possible to reach users who are located at a distance from the library service (Landau, 2010).

SDI by any other name: RSS feeds

SDI is a service that healthcare professionals have provided for many decades, particularly in healthcare, and using computer systems to collate or deliver it is well established (Wood and Seeds, 1974). RSS represents one of the most recent and time-efficient ways to provide this to end-users.

There is some debate about what RSS stands for: it has been variously reported as standing for Rich Site Summary, Report Summary Service, Ready for Some Stories and, more commonly, Really Simple Syndication. RSS provides internet feeds, relaying new information that has been added to a website without the need to set up e-mail alerts. The feeds themselves are coded web pages, designed, in their original form, to be computer readable.

To view most RSS feeds, a news reader or aggregator is required. This software checks the feeds, allowing users to read any newly added content. Some feeds are accessed using a browser; some require downloadable software which may store a copy of the information on a local computer drive.

Many medical and academic journals now incorporate RSS feeds into their websites to alert users to new tables of contents and other editorial additions (Napolitani, 2009).

Looking after the pennies: the cost-effectiveness of Web 2.0

In terms of cost-effectiveness, Web 2.0 applications such as wikis and blogs represent a very cost-effective alternative to buying in web space to, for example, host a website (Robertson et al., 2008). Using Twitter to stay in touch with users, send out publicity notices and alert users to updates at the service is also a far more cost-effective method of communicating with library users than using the old traditional methods of letters or telephone calls, and helps to keep the marketing budget to a minimum. Using wikis or blogs to store documents can also help with storage space, and there are even examples of libraries using Web 2.0 applications as a library management system, notably Koha (www.ptfs-europe.com/?p=797).

All of this must, however, be weighed against the relatively new and unstable nature of hosted Web 2.0-style sites and the tendency of new technology to come and go. Geocities, which hosted tens of thousands of personal websites from the time it was launched in the mid 1990s, closed in 2009, taking with it many personal websites. In 2010 Bloglines, one of the earliest RSS aggregators, also announced that it is to close.

Microblogging

Initially known as a tumblelog, a microblog is a very short, up-to-the-minute message with an instant description of a situation or event. The most famous microblogging application is undoubtedly Twitter, which has rapidly gained in popularity since 2008 (Corbin, 2009). 'Tweets' are the messages users send via text message to their Twitter accounts, appearing on the internet instantaneously. Tweets are limited to just 140 characters. Twitter now offers a real-time alternative to news as portrayed in the traditional media – although admittedly only in small snippets. It has been used to inform the world about Red Cross responses to disasters such as the February 2010 tsunami in Hawaii. It has also been used in some situations to notify rescuers of the whereabouts of possible survivors of disasters and to reassure relatives and friends. Some public health organizations in the USA have also used Twitter to track the spread of diseases such as the flu (http://thenationshealth.aphapublications.org/content/40/8/1.1.full). And, among other uses, Twitter has been used by medical professors to communicate with their students and to send updates from conferences. Other uses include the promotion of an information service (Norman, 2009), which in some cases reaches non-users rather than registered users.

Just as the blogosphere is an overall term for blogs, the twitterverse or twitosphere encompasses Twitter and tweets (Giustini and Wright, 2009).

Let's not forget . . . the user in all of this

Although traditionally healthcare professionals have been somewhat resistant to new technology, the ease of use of the new tools makes it hopeful that this may change in the near future (Brixey and Warren, 2009), although there may be relatively little demand at this early stage for Web 2.0 applications (Ward, Moule and Lockyer, 2009). Where Web 2.0 applications score highly is in enabling users to build communities of practice regardless of what computer they are using.

Much has been written about digital natives, the Millennials or Generation Y, and their level of comfort in an electronic environment. What is, again, very clear is the need for and value of collaborative and group working (Prensky, 2008).

New modes of working: virtual worlds and learning environments

Online role-playing games, precursors of gaming environments like World of Warcraft and virtual worlds like Second Life, were invented in 1979 and were initially known as MUDs (Multi-User Dungeons). Originally entirely text based, MUDs were virtual worlds allowing interaction with others, fiction and online chat. In today's 3D worlds, the user creates an 'avatar', or 3D representative, who can interact with other avatars in the virtual space. Occasionally referred to as MUVEs (multi-user virtual environments), these multi-user worlds have now evolved into virtual locations where users can learn, teach and conduct business affairs, among other activities. Second Life, currently the best known, has already been used for some health education, including at the University of Plymouth and St George's, University of London (Kamel Boulos and Toth-Cohen, 2009).

Other platforms are not virtual worlds, but offer a higher level of interactivity than e-mail or a straightforward video conference call. Many have been specially designed with education and conferencing in mind, such as **Moodle**, **WebEx** and **VoiceThread**; some of them require licensing, some require downloads, and others are free. Some of their potential uses include asynchronous and live learning sessions, conferences or meetings, whether in the same country or as part of an international collaboration.

New skills for new paradigms: the effect on information professionals

The skills that information professionals need in order to thrive in a Web 2.0 world will be changing. Old traditional skills, such as cataloguing, are rapidly being replaced by new, if related, skills such as recording metadata. Catalogues will have to become much more integrated with other tools and applications (Calhoun, 2006), as has already happened in the case of some library management system providers. Innovative Interfaces' Millennium integrated library system, for example, has incorporated Amazon-style recommendations into its Encore facility.

Many library staff have expressed the opinion that their skills to explore and promote Web 2.0 technologies are limited, and that this is compounded by a lack of support from local and central IT development units (Lockyer, Moule and Ward, 2009).

Sneaky teaching

One of the most common applications of Web 2.0 in the medical and healthcare arena is in the realm of education. From nursing to paramedic training, Web 2.0 offers opportunities to deliver and even assess training and education. Podcasts and screencasts offer the option to make education accessible to those who may not be able to attend the live sessions (Kamel Boulos and Wheeler, 2007). St George's, University of London provides an innovative example of a presence in the virtual world Second Life, with the aim of introducing virtual training for paramedics (Hoeksma, 2008).

Truly Miscellaneous

Some Web 2.0 applications defy categorization, like the lovely and somewhat addictive Wordle. Paste a selection of text into the application, and it will return a word picture or cloud, with the term that is repeated most often appearing the largest, and so on, down to the smallest (Figure 2.2). In the health world, Wordle may offer a starting point for analysis of qualitative research or problem-based learning, highlighting major themes for further discussion.

Other applications, such as Animoto, allow the user to upload images and create a short narrative that can then be saved as a video greeting or added to a home page. Others, like MindMeister, offer the option to create collaborative mindmaps; Knol allows the sharing of 'nuggets of knowledge'; and sites such as basecamp offer online

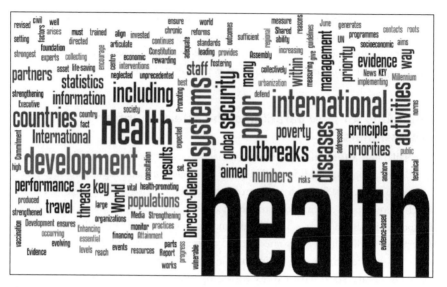

Figure 2.2 *World Health Organisation Agenda, put into Wordle*

project management and file sharing. Other sites such as CalendarHub enable calendar sharing across project teams and different organizations. All of these have potential for use across health organizations.

New applications incorporating image and voice recognition are also beginning to emerge, many specially designed for the iPhone and other mobile devices. Wikitude, for example, is a travel guide that aims to use the information in its database to allow the user to identify, simply via a photograph or image, where they are.

The challenges of Web 2.0

Although the potential for using Web 2.0 in healthcare information is immense, what is lacking as yet is much in-depth analysis of how effective Web 2.0 tools are in delivering healthcare information. There are also relatively few accounts in the academic literature, and what has been written is heavily biased towards education delivery (Kamel Boulos and Wheeler, 2007; McLean, Richards and Wardman, 2007). As with any new technology, Web 2.0 is far from perfect. Major disadvantages include the difficulty of establishing whether the information is authoritative or not, and, in some public sector organizations, the difficulty of accessing the information at all, as firewalls and other security software mean many Web 2.0 applications are blocked.

A disadvantage of Web 2.0, as with all internet sites, is the transience of much of the information. Some excellent blogs, for example, such as http://victormedicina. blogspot.com/ and http://biohealthmatics.blogspot.com/, illustrate this clearly. The posts are very good and informative; but they are several years old and the blogs have not been updated for some time.

Web 2.0 – fad or here to stay?

As with any innovation, doubts have been expressed about whether Web 2.0 is here to stay or is simply a transitory fad. Casual observation of the current generation of students suggests that Web 2.0 applications are here to stay, and, as ever with technology, will evolve rapidly. Web 3.0, or the Semantic Web, is already being discussed in some circles, and is explored later in this book in more detail.

When to use Web 2.0

What isn't always clear is when Web 2.0 can and should be used, or what is the best tool to use. So much depends on personal preferences as often more than one tool is suitable. What is, however, apparent is that the internet is in a constant state of flux, and we are just at the beginning of the journey.

References and further reading

Anderson, P. (2007) What is Web 2.0? Ideas, technologies and implications for education, *JISC Techwatch*, www.jisc.ac.uk/media/documents/techwatch/.

Arthur, C. (2006) What Is the 1% Rule?, *The Guardian*, (20 July), www.guardian.co.uk/technology/2006/jul/20/guardianweeklytechnologysection2.

Bastida, R., Mcgrath, I. and Maude, P. (2010) Wiki Use in Mental Health Practice: recognizing potential use of collaborative technology, *International Journal of Mental Health Nursing*, **19** (2), 142–8.

Billings, D. M. (2009) Wikis and Blogs: consider the possibilities for continuing nursing education, *Journal of Continuing Education in Nursing*, **40** (12), 534–5.

Boulton, C. (2009) *Google Worldwide Search Share Slips a Tad as Queries Soar*, http://bit.ly/9dR9w0.

Boxen, J. L. (2008) Library 2.0: a review of the literature, *The Reference Librarian*, **49** (1), 21–34.

Brixey, J. J. and Warren, J. J. (2009) Creating Experiential Learning Activities Using Web 2.0 Tools and Technologies: a case study, *Studies in Health Technology and Informatics*, **146**, 613–17.

Bryant, S. L., Judkins, T. and Walker, N. (2009) The Commissioning Wiki: an online handbook, *Journal of Management and Marketing in Healthcare*, **2** (3), 305–7.

Bush, V. (1945) As We May Think, *The Atlantic Monthly*, (June), www.theatlantic.com/past/docs/unbound/flashbks/computer/bushf.htm.

Calhoun, K. (2006) *Being a Librarian*, Cornell University Library, http://hdl.handle.net/1813/3561.

Casey, M. E. and Savastinuk, L. C. (2007) Library 2.0: a guide to participatory library service, *Information Today*.

Chad, K. and Miller, P. (2005) *Do Libraries Matter? The rise of Library 2.0*, talis, www.talis.com/applications/downloads/white_papers/DoLibrariesMatter.pdf.

Ciesielka, D. (2008) Using a Wiki to Meet Graduate Nursing Education Competencies in Collaboration and Community Health, *Journal of Nursing Education*, **47** (10), 473–76.

Collins, J. J. (2010) *All About the eBay Sale Experiment*, http://ezinearticles.com/?All-About-the-eBay-Sale-Experiment&id=5412439.

Connor, E. (2008) Using Wiki Technology to Build a Faculty Publications Database, *Journal of Electronic Resources in Medical Libraries*, **4** (4), 11–25.

Corbin, K. (2009) *Twitter Reverses on Reply Tweak After Backlash*, www.internetnews.com/webcontent/article.php/3820256/Twitter+Reverses+on+Reply+Tweak+After+Backlash.htm.

DiNucci, D. (1999) Fragmented Future, *Print*, **53** (4), 32–5, www.cdinucci.com/Darcy2/articles/Print/Printarticle7.html.

Dittems (2008) *The Difference between Web1.0 and Web2.0*, (16 April), http://dittems.blogspot.com/2008/04/difference-between-web10-and-web20.html.

Ebersbach, A., Glaser, M. and Heigl, R. (2006) *Wiki: web collaboration*, Springer-Verlag.

Eysenbach, A. (2008) Medicine 2.0: social networking, collaboration, participation, apomediation, and openness, *Journal of Medical Internet Research*, **10** (3), e22, www.jmir.org/2008/3/e22/.

Gavgani, V. Z. and Mohan, V. V. (2008) Application of Web 2.0 Tools in Medical Librarianship to Support Medicine 2.0, *Webology*, **5** (1), www.webology.ir/2008/v5n1/a53.html.

Giles, J. (2005) Internet Encylopedias go Head to Head, *Nature*, **438**, (7070) 9000–9001.

Giustini, D. (2006) How Web 2.0 Is Changing Medicine, *BMJ*, **333**, 1283–4.

Giustini, D. and Wright, M. D. (2009) Twitter: an introduction to microblogging for health librarians, *Journal of the Canadian Health Libraries Association*, **30**, 11–17.

Guy, M. (2006) Wiki or Won't He? A tale of public sector wikis, *Ariadne*, **49**, www.ariadne.ac.uk/issue49/guy/.

Harris, S. T. and Zeng, X. (2008) Using Wiki in an Online Record Documentation Systems Course, *Perspectives in Health Information Management*, **5** (1), Winter, www.ncbi.nlm.nih.gov/pmc/articles/PMC2242345/pdf/phim0005-0001.pdf.

Healthcare Information for All (2009) *Healthcare Information for All by 2015*, HIFA 2015, www.hifa2015.org/.

Hilska-Keinänen, K. (2009) Wiki as an Intranet, *Journal of the European Association for Health Information and Libraries*, **5** (2), 6–7.

Hinchcliffe, D. (2006) *All We Got Was Web 1.0, when Tim Berners-Lee actually Gave Us Web 2.0*, http://web2.socialcomputingjournal.com/all_we_got_was_web_10_when_tim_bernerslee_actually_gave_us_w.htm.

Hoeksma, J. (2008) *Paramedic students trained using Second Life, e-health insider*, 20 October 2008, www.e-health-insider.com/news/4250/paramedic_students_trained_using_second_life.

Hughes, B., Joshi, I. and Wareham, J. (2008) Health 2.0 and Medicine 2.0: tensions and controversies in the field, *Journal of Medical Internet Research*, **10** (3), e23, http://www.jmir.org/2008/3/e23/.

Kamel Boulos, M. N. and Toth-Cohen, S. (2009) The University of Plymouth Sexual Health Sim Experience in Second Life-®: evaluation and reflections after 1 year, *Health Information and Libraries Journal*, **26** (4), 279–88.

Kamel Boulos, M. N. and Wheeler, S. (2007) The Emerging Web 2.0 Social Software: an enabling suite of sociable technologies in health and healthcare education, *Health Information and Libraries Journal,*, **24** (1), 2–23.

Kamel Boulos, M. N., Maramba, I. and Wheeler, S. (2006) Wikis, Blogs and Podcasts: a new generation of web-based tools for virtual collaborative clinical practice and education, *BMC Medical Education*, **6** (41), www.biomedcentral.com/content/pdf/1472-6920-6-41.pdf.

Kardong-Edgren, S. E., Oermann, M. H., Ha, Y., Tennant, M. N., Snelson, C., Hallmark, E., Rogers, N. and Hurd, D. (2009) Using a Wiki in Nursing Education and Research, *International Journal of Nursing Education Scholarship*, **6** (1), 1–10.

Keast, D. (2009) *The Loneliness of the Long-distance Blogger: using blogs to reach isolated rural health professionals*, http://espace.library.uq.edu.au/eserv/UQ:180024/ n4_1_Thurs_Keast_part2.pdf.

Kent, P. G. (2008) Enticing the Google Generation: Web 2.0, social networking and university students, *29th Annual IATUL Conference*, 21–24 April 2008, Auckland, New Zealand, http://eprints.vu.edu.au/800/1/Kent_P_080201_FINAL.pdf.

Kraft, M. A. (2010) Getting Wiki with It: using a wiki as a web site for regional health system libraries, *Journal of Hospital Librarianship*, **10** (3), 265–78.

Landau, R. (2010) Solo Librarian and Outreach to Hospital Staff Using Web 2.0 Technologies, *Medical Reference Services Quarterly*, **29** (1), 75–84.

Laudon, K. C. and Laudon, J. P. (2001) *Essentials of Management Information Systems*, Pearson Education.

LeFebvre, C. (2009) Integrating cell phones and mobile technologies into public health practice: a social marketing perspective, *Health Promotion Practice*, **10** (4), 490–4.

Lizarondo, L., Kumar, S. and Grimmer-Somers, K. (2010) Online Journal Clubs: an innovative approach to achieving evidence-based practice, *Journal of Allied Health*, **39** (1), e17–22.

MacIntyre, B. (2009), English Acquires its Millionth Word, *Times Online*, 11 June 2009, www.timesonline.co.uk/tol/life_and_style/education/article6475123.ece.

Maness, J. M. (2006) Library 2.0 Theory: Web 2.0 and its implications for libraries, *Webology*, www.webology.ir/2006/v3n2/a25.html?q=link:webology.ir/.

McLean, R., Richards, B. H. and Wardman, J. I. (2007) The Effect of Web 2.0 on the Future of Medical Practice and Education: darwikinian evolution or folksonomic revolution, *The Medical Journal of Australia*, **187** (3), 174–7.

McNab, C. (2009) What Social Media Offers to Health Professionals and Citizens, *Bulletin of The World Health Organisation*, **87**, 566.

Meenan, C., King, A., Toland, C., Daly, M. and Nagy, P. (2010) Use of a Wiki as a Radiology Departmental Knowledge Management System, *Journal of Digital Imaging*, **23** (2), 142–51.

Napolitani, F. (2009) RSS Feed Applications in Libraries: a brief note, *Journal of the European Association for Health Information and Libraries*, **5** (2), 8–9.

Naughton, J. (2006) Websites that Changed the World, *The Guardian*, (13 August), www.guardian.co.uk/technology/2006/aug/13/observerreview.onlinesupplement.

Norman, F. (2009) Using Twitter to Promote Your Institution, *Journal of the European Association for Health Information and Libraries*, **5** (4), 40–2.

O'Reilly, T. (2005) *What Is Web 2.0?: design patterns and business models for the next generation of software*, (30 September), http://oreilly.com/web2/archive/what-is-web-20.html.

O'Reilly, T. and Battelle, J. (2009) *Web Squared: Web 2.0 five years on*, http://assets.en.oreilly.com/1/event/28/web2009_websquared-whitepaper.pdf.

Obst, O. (2008) Using a Wiki for the Library, *Journal of the European Association for Health Information and Libraries*, **4** (2), 50–2, www.eahil.net/journal/journal_2008_vol4_n2.pdf.

Obst, O. (2009) Twitter Reloaded, *Journal of the European Association for Health Information and Libraries*, **5** (3), 45–6.

Pho, K. (2009) *Wikipedia Isn't Really the Patient's Friend*, www.kevinmd.com/blog/2009/08/op-ed-wikipedia-isnt-really-the-patients-friend.html.

Prensky, M. (2008) The Role of Technology in Teaching and the Classroom, *Educational Technology*, Nov-Dec 2008, www.marcprensky.com/writing/Prensky-The_Role_of_Technology-ET-11-12-08.pdf.

Richardson, W. (2005–6) The Educator's Guide to the Read/Write Web, *Educational Leadership*, **63** (4), 24–7.

Robertson, J., Burnham, J., Jie, L. and Sayed, E. (2008) The Medical Matters Wiki: building a library web site 2.0, *Medical Reference Services Quarterly*, **27** (1), 21–32.

Rothman (2009) *List of Medical Wikis*, http://davidrothman.net/list-of-medical-wikis/.

Sharma, P. (2009), *The 'Hotmail' Evolution*, www.techpluto.com/hotmail-evolution/.

Spool, J. (2007) Web 2.0: the power behind the hype, *User Interface Engineering*, (7 August), www.uie.com/articles/web_2_power/.

Surowiecki, J. (2004) *The Wisdom of Crowds*, Little Brown.

Ward, R., Moule, P. and Lockyer, L. (2009) Adoption of Web 2.0 Technologies in Education for Health Professionals in the UK: Where are we and why?, *Journal of Electronic Learning*, **7** (2), 165–172, http://www.ejel.org/issue/download.html?idArticle=151.

Wikipedia (2009) *GeoCities*, http://en.wikipedia.org/wiki/GeoCities (last accessed 13 June 2010).

Wikipedia (2010) *Health 2.0*, http://en.wikipedia.org/wiki/Health_2.0 (last accessed 13 June 2010).

Wood, M. S. and Seeds, R. S. (1974) Development of SDI Services from a Manual

Current Awareness Service to SDILINE, *Bulletin of the Medical Library Association*, **62** (4), 374–84.

Wootton, R., Patil, N. G. and Ho, K. (2009) *Telehealth in the Developing World*, Royal Society of Medicine Press.

World Bank (2010) *World Development Indicators*, http://data.worldbank.org/sites/default/files/wdi-final.pdf.

PART 2

Web 2.0 and the implications for health information

CHAPTER 3

Emerging technologies in health, medical and nursing education

Patricia Anderson

Introduction

Appropriate use of online technologies in healthcare education can reduce costs, maximize utility of scarce resources, as well as extend temporal and geographic access to educational content. Those factors alone would serve as valid justification for exploring their use; however, there is more. Online social environments can provide access to educational experiences that are not possible or ethical in face-to-face environments, can extend access to patient communities, and can actually provide new and enriched therapeutic and support environments for both education and clinical practice. Being aware of new and emerging uses of technology in healthcare and having the practical skills to stay current in these areas are no longer optional or a nicety. Rather, they are essential for clinicians of the future, who will require this knowledge in order to remain functional in evolving clinical practice and to communicate efficiently and credibly with certain patient populations.

The use of emerging technologies in healthcare education has particular relevance in addressing the recent Carnegie Report observation that 'learners have inadequate opportunities to work with patients over time and to observe the course of illness and recovery; students and residents often poorly understand non-clinical physician roles' (Cooke, Irby and O'Brien, 2010). Simulations, virtual reality and virtual worlds are particularly valuable in addressing the latter, while social technologies and mobile applications are especially well suited for the former. Gaming and serious games can be applied in both of these environments as well as many others, depending on the design and intent of the program. In this chapter, several major online educational technologies will be reviewed for their application to healthcare education, with specific examples provided to illustrate their use.

Emerging technologies in education

Instead, by apprenticeship we mean a range of integrative learning required for any professional that includes (1) instantiating, articulating, and making visible and accessible key aspects of competent and expert performance; (2) giving learners a chance for supervised practice; (3) coaching in the supervised practice to help students understand, reflect on, and articulate their practice, particularly the nature of particular clinical situations; (4) helping novice students recognize the priorities and demands embedded in particular clinical situations so that they gain a sense of salience, that is, what must be attended to and addressed in relation to the significance and urgency in the particular clinical situation; and (5) reflection on practice to help the student develop a self-improving practice. (Benner et al., 2009, 25–6)

Emerging technologies in education focus primarily on those technologies that allow collaboration between teachers and students and engagement with content, such as blogging, wikis, social media of all sorts, games, simulations and virtual worlds, and mashups of the various options, so as to create novel interfaces to content. The Horizon Report from the New Media Consortium has become a leading tool in identifying new technologies for education, both those currently being used and those that are newly arising (Johnson et al., 2010).

Emerging technologies in healthcare cover a range of topics, from augmented reality (AR) to YouTube, with robotics, games, simulations and virtual reality along the way. A detailed search in December 2009 on PubMed for 'emerging technologies' found 1636 articles, of which over a quarter (28%) had to do with virtual reality (VR), virtual worlds (VW) and Second Life (SL) (Figure 3.1). When the search was limited to use in healthcare education, the percentage was even higher (45%, n=323). A search in the primary educational research database, ERIC, did not allow searching for the broad term 'Web 2.0', but otherwise showed generally similar patterns per topic, for example returning 1695 citations (December 2009) for the same three concepts of VR/VW/SL, clearly showing that VW and VR are no longer truly new concepts in education (Figure 3.2).

In both education and healthcare, educational simulations appear in thousands of articles and are plainly well established, with simulations having been used in medical education and nursing since the 1960s (Clark, 1976; Clark, 1977; Issenberg et al., 2005; Nehring and Lashley, 2009; Rosen, 2008). What is new is not the idea of simulations but, rather, creating simulations in online spaces, using VR and VW. Emerging technologies appear throughout healthcare education in a diversity of subject domains (see Appendix to this chapter). Technologies currently of greatest interest in healthcare education include serious games, mobile technologies and smartphones, simulations of various types, virtual reality, virtual worlds and the broad category of social technologies often referred to as 'Web 2.0'. Serious games, as a concept, range from educational games in a curricular context to games for a purpose – education, outreach, activism, awareness, behaviour change, problem solving, crowdsourcing and more – within the broader society.

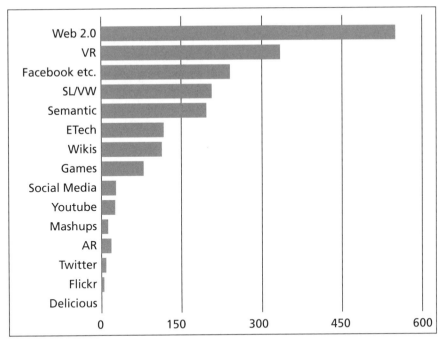

Figure 3.1 *Results of PubMed search on 'emerging technologies', December 2009 (n=1636)*

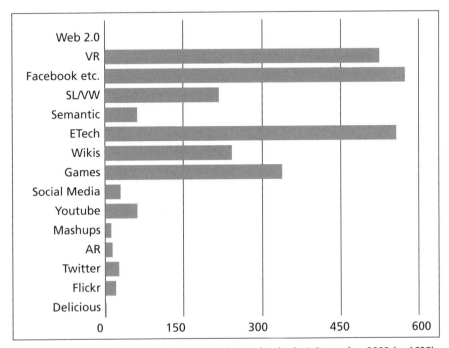

Figure 3.2 *Results of ERIC search on 'emerging technologies', December 2009 (n=1695)*

Serious games

Reviews of the research agree that, as with most emerging or innovative educational approaches, there is not enough evidence at this time to confirm the superiority of the innovation, but that anecdotal evidence supports enthusiasm. Susi et al. (2007) justify the domain with economics, relating serious games to 'e-learning, edutainment, game-based learning, and digital game-based learning', and questioning designs that do not promote critical thinking along with engagement. Critical thinking is also identified as being significant by Brown and Chronister (2009), who provide an example of a simulation design that succeeds in producing this. Susi et al. (2007) also justify games as a way to position learning within a relevant and appropriate context, a justification that is especially apt when extended to VR and VW. Foreman et al. (2004) place serious games in the context of existing imperfections in current instructional models, reasoning that it is worth trying new approaches when the current approaches fail to reach their desired goals.

In healthcare, there have been two Cochrane systematic reviews of serious games. Bhoopathi and Sheoran (2006) evaluated games for training mental health professionals, and found that there was insufficient evidence, despite consistent positive effect. Akl et al. (2008b) likewise found insufficient evidence, warning potential developers to seriously consider the advantages (positive perception, improved communication, team building and collaboration) and disadvantages (development, costs, times, assessment) of games. Blakely et al. (2009), in their systematic review of education gaming in healthcare, explicitly extended the discussion of advantages and disadvantages into a comparison with traditional didactic instruction, including issues related to perceived stress and anxiety and enriching issues related to evaluation.

3D technologies

> Current 3D learning technologies are simply the natural extension and convergence of several technologies currently used for online learning. The converging technologies are synchronous learning tools, Web 2.0, social networking, and video games. ... The environment can be realistic, like a classroom, or it can be surreal, like the creation of a giant computer, drill, or the inside of an artery. (Kapp and O'Driscoll, 2010, 344)

VW and VR are most used in education for their qualities of immersiveness, presence, engagement, portability and relative effectiveness. In general, they extend the 'learning-by-doing' and apprenticeship models from the effective but very expensive and sometimes risky or unfeasible face-to-face mode of learning into spaces that 'help save lives, resources and time' (USC Institute for Creative Technologies, 2010). They also serve as a technology to extend simulations into new spaces.

> Learning-by-doing is generally considered the most effective way to learn. The Internet and

a variety of emerging communication, visualization, and simulation technologies now make it possible to offer students authentic learning experiences ranging from experimentation to real-world problem solving. (Lombardi, 2007)

Lombardi (2007) identifies the most relevant emerging technologies currently applicable to healthcare education, and lists the main types of educational concerns for which they are best suited:

1 Real-world relevance
2 Ill-defined problem
3 Sustained investigation
4 Multiple sources and perspectives
5 Collaboration
6 Reflection (metacognition)
7 Interdisciplinary perspective
8 Integrated assessment
9 Polished products
10 Multiple interpretations and outcomes.

Of these ten concerns, the most important is real-world relevance, especially in the context given by Lombardi when she says, 'Authentic activities match the real-world tasks of professionals in practice as nearly as possible'. This is echoed by Smith (2009), who states that 'active learning exercises in a clinically realistic setting can improve psychomotor performance, critical-thinking decision making, clinician confidence, professional satisfaction, and interpersonal team skills'. Oddsson et al. (2007), in their research on using VR for rehabilitation for balance disorders, confirmed the potential for psychomotor performance improvements, implying that somatosensory cues in VR can create true immersive experiences. George and De (2010) discuss effective use of VR for replacing cadaveric dissection in training, saving costs and addressing scarcity of resources and time constraints. Kaphingst et al. (2009a) found VR environments similar to SL, appropriate for building communication skills, with this important caveat – technology, especially emerging and innovative technologies, can prove a barrier to learning (Kaphingst et al., 2009b). Issenberg et al. (2005) emphasize the need for simulations of any sort to occur in 'a controlled environment where learners can make, detect and correct errors without adverse consequences', listing the following as the core criteria for a successful educational simulation:

1 Educational feedback
2 Repetitive practice
3 Curriculum integration
4 Range of difficulty level
5 Multiple learning strategies

6 Clinical variation
7 Controlled environment
8 Individualized learning
9 Defined outcomes
10 Simulator validity.

A combination of the Lombardi and Issenberg criteria makes a useful set for developing and defining expectations and assessing simulations and the use of emerging technologies in healthcare education.

New trends

Important new trends in simulation and emerging technologies in education include augmented reality, haptics, mobile technologies and smartphones. Educational informatics is a relatively new field tracking these types of trends (Ford, 2004; Levy et al., 2003) that has been rapidly adopted within healthcare education (D'Alessandro and D'Alessandro, 2009; New York University, 2009; Weiner, 2008; Weiner and Tragenstein, 2009). Augmented reality is, simply stated, the use of technology to enhance our perception of the real world with additional information, currently usually either visual or data. In this context, haptics refers to the use of technology to provide sensory input, especially tactile or touch-sensitive feedback. Smartphones include Android, Blackberry, iPhone and others, all of which offer, in addition to cell phone capability, web access and downloadable applications. It is possible and likely that all three of these (AR, haptics and smartphones) will combine for future training and on-site diagnostic/triage support. Botden et al. (2007) compared the combination of AR and haptics to VR simulation for training, finding 'that AR offers better realism, haptic feedback, didactic value, and construct validity than does VR, and it also gives useful feedback to determine trainee skill levels'.

Mobile, smartphone and portable e-book and audio devices have become increasingly important in healthcare education (Ducut and Fontelo, 2008), with uses ranging from podcasts and recorded lectures to flashcards and other self-study tools to research and reference sources to patient simulations and assignments to in-class quizzes. Aside from the many overtly educational uses, mobile devices are also increasingly used in clinical care, research and monitoring and fill other healthcare functions, requiring that they be included in training for clinical practice. Examples of recent health uses of smartphones include telesurgery consultations (Aziz and Ziccardi, 2009), diabetes management (Arsand et al., 2008; Cho et al., 2009), and communication support for persons with autism (De Leo and Leroy, 2008). Extending beyond the immediate, both Aanensen et al. (2009) and Pentland et al. (2009) describe the use of smartphones for harvesting routine data from people simply carrying their phones around to provide both community health and planning data as well as the potential for early diagnosis of significant health conditions.

To date, most of the use of AR in healthcare education has been as an extension to simulations and limited to cumbersome headgear, often called Heads-Up Displays or HUDs. When integrated with haptics, it often involves the use of an even more cumbersome and expensive bodysuit, but has provided highly successful and replicable learning experiences. Examples of recent uses of AR in healthcare education include lab animal-science training (Ketelhut and Niemi, 2007) and suturing training (Botden et al., 2009). A particularly relevant application of AR has been the enrichment of data for healthy, trained, standardized patients so as to model specific disease conditions for an Objective Structured Clinical Examination (OSCE) (McKenzie et al., 2006).

Kinnison et al. (2009) have integrated haptics into anatomy training simulations. The year 2009 saw the first popular AR applications designed for smartphones. Wikitude and Cyclopedia are two AR applications that combine location-sensitivity with Wikipedia data, making it possible to point your phone camera at a building and bring up an article about that location (Kirkpatrick, 2009). Dave deBronkart (2009) asked, 'Why not Google Earth for my body?', while earlier the same year mobile video systems have made it possible for emergency medical service providers to engage emergency department doctors in triage while the ambulance is on its way to the hospital (Versel, 2009).

With AR being combined separately with both haptics and smartphones, it is realistic to anticipate future devices combining these three new technologies in ways that might make it possible to provide a Google Earth-type view of a person on the street or a simulated patient in a realistic scenario, with real-time interaction with remote trainers or clinicians.

Education in Second Life

Education is thriving in Second Life. This enthusiastic subculture is abuzz within the Second Life realm, constantly interacting inside and outside Second Life. Educators are exploring every possible tool the 3D virtual world offers and establishing best practices along the way. (Harrison, 2009)

The first educators in SL taught courses on art, architecture, business, instructional technology, urban planning, human–computer interface, communities, sociology, education, game design, healthcare and disaster response, and simulation development (Linden, 2005). The earliest articles in the professional education literature specifically about SL date from 2006, about a year after educators began teaching in SL. They included articles about a schizophrenia simulation (Yellowlees and Cook, 2006), educational technologies (Delwiche, 2006) and role-playing (Childress and Braswell, 2006). Early strengths identified in working with the SL platform specifically and VW in general included rapport, immersiveness and communication (Gratch et al., 2007), as well as access to objects, environments and people normally inaccessible in real time (Strangman and Hall, 2003). These real-time barriers to access can be logistical or physical, such as simulation rooms inaccessible after 5.00 pm, or they may be social or ethical in nature, such as learning patient care and problem-solving skills in situations or for populations that involve protected populations or high risk. Communication skills (Jarmon et al., 2009), social and language learning have continued to be areas in which SL education has been shown to excel. Previous educational efforts within the local campus SL community included small group projects, lectures, research presentations, disaster simulations, invited speakers, tours, credit courses (ranging from Italian to pharmacy), skills workshops, conferences and immersive games (Anderson and Stephens, 2008; Stephens, 2009).

While education is probably the leading non-recreational use of SL at this time, healthcare has a strong presence, as evidenced by the hundreds of locations, groups and events discoverable in the community-generated wiki SLHealthy (2007–) and the community in the SL group Healthcare Education. A number of more formal publications describe the range and potential of healthcare activities in SL (Kamel Boulos, Hetherington and Wheeler, 2007; Hansen, 2008; Beard et al., 2009). Baker (2009) noted part of the value of serious games as allowing students to 'experience an environment for practice without real harm or risk to patients', something that is perhaps even more possible within the SL immersive experience. Gratch et al. (2007) noted that VW can provide even 'stronger rapport-like effects than face-to-face communication between human partners'. Nelson and Blenkin (2007) noted the powerful presence of education in VW, observing that 'students regarded the role-play environment as a physical building with rooms in which they interacted'.

VW has been found to be effective in education for patients and persons with disabilities – an important factor in providing both distance learning and universal access to learning experiences for special populations (Strangman and Hall, 2003; Krueger et al., 2009). It is these qualities and the presence of a widely varied and international population that make SL so potentially powerful for role-play simulations of healthcare challenges and collaborations.

Healthcare education in SL also stretches beyond role play and simulations. Dr Douglas Danforth (known in SL as DrDoug Pennell) achieved a certain notoriety for building a model of the testes and spermatogenesis as large as a football field (Oleetzel, 2008), while at the Ann Myers Medical Center in SL real doctors and nurses mentor real healthcare students in working with real patients (Dolan, 2008).

Nursing has long been recognized as one of the healthcare communities at the forefront of engaging with SL (Hansen, 2008). Nursing schools active in SL include Duke University (2009), East Carolina University (Corbett et al., 2008), Glasgow Caledonian University (McElhinney, 2009), Imperial College London (Raeside, 2008), University of Auckland, New Zealand (Lafsky, 2009), University of Kansas Medical Center (KUMC) (Gerald and Antonacci, 2009a and 2009b), University of Wisconsin, Green Bay (Wong, 2009) and University of Wisconsin, Oshkosh (Paine, 2009; Schmidt and Stewart, 2009; Skiba, 2009; Stewart et al., 2009). Probably the earliest adopter and most active has been Tacoma Community College, through the leadership of John Miller, who is also a cofounder of MUVErsLLC, the leading developer of sophisticated healthcare simulations in SL (Nursing 211, 2007; Ford and Miller, 2008; Lafsky, 2009; Miller, 2008; Miller, 2009; MUVErsLLC, 2009).

Conclusion

Trends apparent both from the search results and literature review show that social technologies currently take precedence as applications for healthcare education, followed closely by immersive technologies such as VR and VWs. In recent years there has been considerable discussion about the healthcare information explosion and the challenges for practising clinicians in staying current and knowledgeable within their domains of expertise (Davies, 2007). Indeed, these were leading factors in support of the shift towards evidence-based healthcare and the development and refinement of systematic review methodologies.

This pattern is certainly just as true, if not more so, within healthcare education, given that expertise is required not only in healthcare but also in teaching and learning trends and technologies. Discovering new technologies and determining which are most useful and relevant is a significant and sometimes questionable challenge in today's healthcare practice environment (Spallek et al., 2010). Learning new technologies for personal use requires a certain amount of time; developing sufficient competence to use them in teaching requires much more.

Just as, in evidence-based and systematic review methodologies, a critical role for the librarian is to strategically define searching techniques for discovering and tracking trends within a topic over time, so librarians can play a similar role in discovering, tracking and disseminating emerging technologies that have application to healthcare educators and researchers. Just as librarians have supported educators and learners with bibliographic instruction during several generations, so librarians can take a lead role in learning and providing training support in these new educational technologies as they are adopted. Reviews such as this one are only the beginning of how librarians can support healthcare educators in exploring and integrating new technologies into their teaching and practice.

Appendix *Selected examples of emerging technologies in healthcare education*

Reviews/overviews	Gaming	Mobile	Simulations	Virtual reality	Virtual worlds/SL	Web 2.0
	Akl et al. (2008b) Blakely et al. (2009)	Ducut & Fontelo (2008)		Mantovani et al. (2003)	Kamel Boulos, Hetherington & Wheeler (2007)	Kamel Boulos & Wheeler (2007) Hughes et al. (2008)
Medicine	**Gaming**	**Mobile**	**Simulations**	**Virtual reality**	**Virtual worlds/SL**	**Web 2.0**
Anatomy		Trelease (2008)	Kinnison et al. (2009)	George & De (2010)		George & De (2010)
Carotid artery stenting				Berry et al. (2008)		
Clinical practice guidelines	Akl et al. (2008a)					
Communication skills				Kaphingst et al. (2009a)	Zielke et al. (2009)	
Continuing Medical Education	Telner et al. (2010)			Wiecha et al. (2010)		Kamel Boulos, Maramba & Wheeler (2006) Chu et al. (2010) McLean et al. (2007)
Dental			Eaton et al. (2008)	Eaton et al. (2008)	Phillips & Berge (2009) Eaton et al. (2008)	Mattheos et al. (2008)
Dermatology						Vance et al. (2009)
Diabetes		Arsand et al. (2008) Cho et al. (2009)				
Disabilities					Krueger, Ludwig & Ludwig (2009) Zielke et al. (2009)	
Emergency preparation, triage, critical care simulations	Bergeron (2008)		Bergeron (2008) Lamb (2007)	Bergeron (2008)	Ramloll et al. (2006)	
Genetic literacy				Kaphingst et al. (2009a)		
Geriatric house calls, long-term care	Duque et al. (2008)		Nelson & Blenkin (2007)		Nelson & Blenkin (2007)	
Global health						
Gynaecological endoscopy				Mettler & Dewan (2009)		
Laboratory animal science	Ketelhut & Niemi (2007)		Ketelhut & Niemi (2007)	Ketelhut & Niemi (2007)	Ketelhut & Niemi (2007)	
Laparoscopic & endoscopic training			Snyder et al. (2009)	Snyder et al. (2009)		

Appendix (*Continued*)

Medicine (Continued)	Gaming	Mobile	Simulations	Virtual reality	Virtual worlds/SL	Web 2.0
Obstetric emergencies		Deering et al. (2009)		Deering et al. (2009)		
Pathology						Schreiber & Giustini (2009) Wick (2009)
Patient communication, education & safety			Smith (2009)	Kaphingst et al. (2009a)	Kamel Boulos & Toth-Cohen (2009)	
Pharmacology						Cain & Fox (2009)
Radiology	Reiner & Siegel (2008)					
Regional anesthesia				Grottke et al. (2009)		
Rehabilitation		Svoboda & Richards (2009)		Oddsson et al. (2007)		
Research skills						Anderson et al. (2009)
Surgery & telesurgery		Russomano et al. (2009) Aziz & Ziccardi (2009)	Gamboa et al. (2009)	Russomano et al. (2009)		
Suturing			Botden et al. (2009)			
Nursing	Gaming	Mobile	Simulations	Virtual reality	Virtual worlds/SL	Web 2.0
Nursing	Barber & Norman (1989)				Walker et al. (2009) Hansen (2008)	Lemley & Burnham (2009)
Airway management			Cason et al. (2010)			
Education	Royse & Newton (2007) Skiba et al. (2008)	Skiba et al. (2008)	Morrison et al. (2009) Skiba et al. (2008)		Skiba et al. (2008)	Skiba et al. (2008) Burke et al. (2009)
Electrocardiogram			Brown & Chronister (2009)			
End-of-life care			Leighton & Dubas (2009)			
Pediatric			Butler et al. (2009)			

Appendix *(Continued)*

Nursing *(Continued)*	Gaming	Mobile	Simulations	Virtual reality	Virtual worlds/SL	Web 2.0
Perioperative nursing	Baker (2009) Smith (2009)			Smith (2009)	Gerald & Antonacci (2009a) Gerald & Antonacci (2009b)	
Renal care	Foster & Dallemagne (2009)				Foster & Dallemagne (2009)	
Psychology and psychiatry	**Gaming**	**Mobile**	**Simulations**	**Virtual reality**	**Virtual worlds/SL**	**Web 2.0**
Addiction				Virtually Better (2009)		
Clinical psychiatry					Gorini et al. (2008)	
Mental health	Bhoopathi & Sheoran (2006)				Walker (2009)	
Phobias				Virtually Better (2009)		
PTSD (general, Iraq & Vietnam)				Rothbaum et al. (2001) Virtually Better (2009)	Gerardi et al. (2008) Reger et al. (2009) Reger & Gahm (2008) Rizzo et al. (2009) Rizzo et al. (2008) Rizzo et al. (2005) Walker (2009) Wood et al. (2009)	
Public health	**Gaming**	**Mobile**	**Simulations**	**Virtual reality**	**Virtual worlds/SL**	**Web 2.0**
Public health						Vance et al. (2009)
GIS		Kamel Boulos, Scotch, Cheung & Burden (2008)	Kamel Boulos, Scotch, Cheung & Burden (2008)		Kamel Boulos, Scotch, Cheung & Burden (2008) Boulos & Burden (2007)	Kamel Boulos, Scotch, Cheung & Burden (2008)
Global health						Maru et al. (2009)
Modelling HIV/AIDS		Aanensen et al. (2009)			Gordon et al. (2009)	
Modelling epidemics/communities					Lofgren & Fefferman (2007)	
Occupational and environmental					Kamel Boulos, Ramloll, Jones & Toth-Cohen (2008)	

References

Aanensen, D. M., Huntley, D. M., Feil, E. J., al-Own, F. and Spratt, B. G. (2009) EpiCollect: linking smartphones to web applications for epidemiology, ecology and community data collection, *PLoS One*, **4** (9), e6968, www.plosone.org/article/info:doi/10.1371/journal.pone.0006968.

Akl, E. A., Mustafa, R., Slomka, T., Alawneh, A., Vedavalli, A. and Schünemann, H. J. (2008a) An Educational Game for Teaching Clinical Practice Guidelines to Internal Medicine Residents: development, feasibility and acceptability, *BMC Medical Education*, **18** (8), 50, www.biomedcentral.com/1472-6920/8/50.

Akl, E. A., Sackett, K., Pretorius, R., Erdley, S., Bhoopathi, P. S., Mustafa, R. and Schünemann, H. J. (2008b) Educational Games for Health Professionals, *Cochrane Database of Systematic Reviews*, **23** (1), CD006411.

Anderson, P. F. and Stephens, M. (2008) Wolverine Island, *EDUCAUSE Review*, **43** (5), supplement, www.educause.edu/EDUCAUSE+Review/ EDUCAUSEReviewMagazineVolume43/WolverineIsland/163175.

Anderson, P. F., Blumenthal, J., Bruell, D., Rosenzweig, M., Conte, M. and Song, J. (2009) An Online and Social Media Training Curricula to Facilitate Bench-to-Bedside Information Transfer. Presented at *Positioning the Profession: the Tenth International Congress on Medical Librarianship*, Brisbane Australia, 31 August–4 September, http://espace.library.uq.edu.au/view/UQ:179795.

Arsand, E., Tufano, J. T., Ralston, J. D. and Hjortdahl, P. (2008) Designing Mobile Dietary Management Support Technologies for People with Diabetes, *Journal of Telemed Telecare*, **14** (7), 329–32.

Aziz, S. R. and Ziccardi, V. B. (2009) Telemedicine Using Smartphones for Oral and Maxillofacial Surgery Consultation, Communication, and Treatment Planning, *Journal of Oral and Maxillofacial Surgery*, **67** (11), 2505–9.

Baker, J. D. (2009) Serious games and perioperative nursing, *AORN Journal*, **90** (2), 173–5.

Barber, P. and Norman, I. (1989) Preparing Teachers for the Performance and Evaluation of Gaming-simulation in Experiential Learning Climates, *Journal of Advanced Nursing*, **14** (2), 146–51.

Beard, L., Wilson, K., Morra, D. and Keelan, J. (2009) A Survey of Health-related Activities on Second Life, *Journal of Medical Internet Research*, 22, **11** (2), e17, www.jmir.org/2009/2/e17/HTML.

Benner, P., Sutphen, M., Leonard, V. and Day, L. (2009) *Educating Nurses: a call for radical transformation* (The Carnegie Foundation for the Advancement of Teaching), Jossey-Bass, www.josseybass.com/WileyCDA/WileyTitle/ productCd-0470457961,descCd-description.html.

Bergeron, B. P. (2008) Learning and Retention in Adaptive Serious Games, *Studies in Health Technology and Informatics*, **132**, 26–30.

Berry, M., Reznick, R., Lystig, T. and Lönn, L. (2008) The Use of Virtual Reality for Training in Carotid Artery Stenting: a construct validation study, *Acta Radiologica*, **49** (7), 801–5.

Bhoopathi, P. S. and Sheoran, R. (2006) Educational Games for Mental Health Professionals, *Cochrane Database of Systematic Reviews*, **19** (2), CD001471.

Blakely, G., Skirton, H., Cooper, S., Allum, P. and Nelmes, P. (2009) Educational Gaming in the Health Sciences: systematic review, *Journal of Advanced Nursing*, **65** (2), 259–69.

Botden, S. M. B. I., Buzink, S. N., Schijven, M. P. and Jakimowicz, J. J. (2007) Augmented versus Virtual Reality Laparoscopic Simulation: what is the difference? A comparison of the ProMIS augmented reality laparoscopic simulator versus LapSim virtual reality laparoscopic simulator, *World Journal of Surgery*, **31**, 764–772.

Botden, S. M. B. I., de Hingh, I. H. J. T. and Jakimowicz, J. J. (2009) Suturing Training in Augmented Reality: gaining proficiency in suturing skills faster, *Surgical Endoscopy*, **23**, 2131–2137.

Brown, D. and Chronister, C. (2009) The Effect of Simulation Learning on Critical Thinking and Self-confidence when Incorporated into an Electrocardiogram Nursing Course, *Clinical Simulation in Nursing*, **5**, e45-e52.

Burke, S. C., Snyder, S. and Rager, R. C. (2009) An Assessment of Faculty Usage of YouTube as a Teaching Resource, *Internet Journal of Allied Health Sciences and Practice*, **7** (1), http://ijahsp.nova.edu/articles/Vol7Num1/burke.htm.

Butler, K. W., Veltre, D. E. and Brady, D. (2009) Implementation of Active Learning Pedagogy Comparing Low-Fidelity Simulation Versus High-Fidelity Simulation in Pediatric Nursing Education, *Clinical Simulation in Nursing*, **5**, e129–e136.

Cain, J. and Fox, B. I. (2009) Web 2.0 and Pharmacy Education, *American Journal of Pharmacy Education*, **73** (7), Article 120.

Cason, C. L., Cazzell, M. A., Nelson, K. A., Hartman, V., Roye, J. and Mancini, M. E. (2010) Improving Learning of Airway Management with Case-based Computer Microsimulations, *Clinical Simulation in Nursing*, **6**, e15–e23.

Childress, M. D. and Braswell, R. (2006) Using Massively Multiplayer Online Role-Playing Games for Online Learning, *Distance Education*, **27** (2), 187–196.

Cho, J. H., Lee, H. C., Lim, D. J., Kwon, H. S. and Yoon, K. H. (2009) Mobile Communication Using a Mobile Phone with a Glucometer for Glucose Control in Type 2 Patients with Diabetes: as effective as an internet-based glucose monitoring system, *Journal of Telemedicine and Telecare*, **15** (2), 77–82.

Chu, L.F., Young, C., Zamora, A., Kurup, V. and Macario, A. (2010) Anesthesia 2.0: internet-based information resources and Web 2.0 applications in anesthesia education, *Current Opinion in Anaesthesiology*, April, **23** (2), 218–27, http://journals.lww.com/co-anesthesiology/Abstract/2010/04000/Anesthesia_2_0__Internet_based_information.16.aspx.

Clark, C. (1977) Learning Outcomes in a Simulation Game for Associate Degree Nursing Students, *Health Education Monographs*, **5** (suppl. 1), 18–27.

Clark, C. C. (1976) Simulation Gaming: a new teaching strategy in nursing education, *Nurse Education*, **1** (4), 4–9.

Cooke, M., Irby, D. M. and O'Brien, B. C. (2010) *A Summary of Educating Physicians: a call for reform of medical school and residency*, Carnegie Foundation for the Advancement of Teaching, www.carnegiefoundation.org/elibrary/summary-educating-physicians.

Corbett, R. W., Sessoms, A., Green, B. and Chen, K. (2008) Second Life 'Note Cards' in the College of Nursing. Presented at East Carolina University's *The Virtual Worlds in Education Conference*, (10–11 November), https://team.nursing.ecu.edu/conexchange/faculty/MeetFacultyStaff/Undergra duateFaculty/BobGreen/SecondLifeConference/tabid/546/Default.aspx.

D'Alessandro, D. M. and D'Alessandro, M. P. (2004–2009) EducationalInformatics.org, a Laboratory for the Study of Educational Informatics, *EducationalInformatics.org*, www.educationalinformatics.org/.

Davies, K. (2007) The Information-seeking Behaviour of Doctors: a review of the evidence, *Health Information and Libraries Journal*, **24**, 78–94.

De Leo, G. and Leroy, G. (2008) An Online Community for Teachers of Children with Autism to Support, Observe, and Evaluate Communication Enabled with Smartphones, *AMIA Annual Symposium Proceedings*, **6**, 924.

deBronkart, D. (ePatientDave) (2009) 'The Quantified Patient': my talk at 'Quantified Self', *ePatients.net*, (December 27), http://e-patients.net/archives/2009/12/the-quantified-patient-my-talk-at-quantified-self-showtell-december-2009.html.

Deering, S., Rosen, M. A., Salas, E. and King, H. B. (2009) Building Team and Technical Competency for Obstetric Emergencies: the mobile obstetric emergencies simulator (MOES) system, *Simulation in Healthcare*, **4** (3), 166–73.

Delwiche, A. (2006) Massively Multiplayer Online Games (MMOs) in the New Media Classroom, *Journal of Educational Technology & Society*, **9** (3), 160–172.

Dolan, P. L. (2008) Parallel Universe: entering an online 3-D world, the medical community is trying to find real-life benefits from the virtual reality of Second Life, *American Medical News*, (8 September), www.ama-assn.org/amednews/2008/09/08/bisa0908.htm.

Ducut, E. and Fontelo, P. (2008) Mobile Devices in Health Education: current use and practice, *Journal of Computing in Higher Education*, **20**, 59–68.

Duke University School of Nursing (2009) *DUSON Second Life*, http://nursing.duke.edu/modules/son_about/index.php?id=90.

Duque, G., Fung, S., Mallet, L., Posel, N. and Fleiszer, D. (2008) Learning while Having Fun: the use of video gaming to teach geriatric house calls to medical students, *Journal of the American Geriatrics Society*, **56** (7), 1328–32.

Eaton, K. A., Reynolds, P. A., Grayden, S. K. and Wilson, N. H. F. (2008) A Vision of Dental Education in the Third Millennium, *British Dental Journal*, **205** (5), 261–271, www.haptel.kcl.ac.uk/wordpress/wp-content/uploads/2009/09/Eaton-Reynolds-Grayden-and-Wilson-2008.pdf.

Ford, N. (2004) Towards a Model of Learning for Educational Informatics, *Journal of Documentation*, **60** (2), 183–225.

Ford, S. and Miller, J. (2008) Simulation and Teaching in Second Life. Presented at *Best Practices in Allied Health/Health Sciences*, Renton Technical Community College, 7 May, www.slideshare.net/jsvavoom/best-practices-renton-conf-may-7-2008.

Foreman, J., Gee, J. P., Herz, J. C., Hinrichs, R. and Prensky, M. (2004) Game-Based Learning: how to delight and instruct in the 21st century, *EDUCAUSE Review*, **39** (5), 50–66.

Foster, J. and Dallemagne, C. (2009) Teaching Undergraduate Nursing Students Renal Care in a 3D Gaming Environment, *Studies in Health Technology and Informatics*, **146**, 837–40.

Gamboa, A. J. R., Box, G. N., Preminger, G. M. and McDougall, E. M. (2009) NOTES: Education and training, *Journal of Endourology*, **23** (5), 813–819.

George, A. P. and De, R. (2010) Review of Temporal Bone Dissection Teaching: how it was, is and will be, *Journal of Laryngology & Otology*, **124** (2), 119–25.

Gerald, S. and Antonacci, D. M. (2009a) Teaching Nurse Anesthesia in a Second Life Operating Room Simulation, *EDUCAUSE Annual Conference*, (29 October), www.educause.edu/Resources/TeachingNurseAnesthesiainaSeco/163388.

Gerald, S. and Antonacci, D. M. (2009b) Virtual World Learning Spaces: developing a Second Life operating room simulation, *EDUCAUSE Quarterly*, **32** (1), www.educause.edu/EDUCAUSE+Quarterly/EDUCAUSEQuarterlyMagazineVolum/VirtualWorldLearningSpacesDeve/163851.

Gerardi, M., Rothbaum, B. O., Ressler, K., Heekin, M. and Rizzo, A. (2008) Virtual Reality Exposure Therapy Using a Virtual Iraq: case report, *Journal of Trauma Stress*, **21** (2), 209–13.

Gordon, R., Björklund, N. K., Smith, R. J. and Blyden, E. R. (2009) Halting HIV/AIDS with Avatars and Havatars: a virtual world approach to modelling epidemics, *BMC Public Health*, **9** (suppl. 1), S13.

Gorini, A., Gaggioli, A., Vigna, C. and Riva, G. (2008) A Second Life for eHealth: prospects for the use of 3-D virtual worlds in clinical psychology, *Journal of Medical Internet Research*, **10** (3), e21.

Gratch, J., Wang, N., Okhmatovskaia, A., Lamothe, F., Morales, M., van der Werf, R. J. and Morency, L. P. (2007) Can Virtual Humans Be more Engaging than Real Ones? *12th International Conference on Human-Computer Interaction*, Beijing, China, http://ict.usc.edu/files/publications/HCI07.pdf.

Grottke, O., Ntouba, A., Ullrich, S., Liao, W., Fried, E., Prescher, A., Deserno, T. M., Kuhlen, T. and Rossaint, R. (2009) Virtual Reality-based Simulator for Training in Regional Anaesthesia, *British Journal of Anaesthesia*, **103** (4), 594–600.

Hansen, M. M. (2008) Versatile, Immersive, Creative and Dynamic Virtual 3-D Healthcare Learning Environments: a review of the literature, *Journal of Medical Internet Research*, **10** (3), e26.

Harrison, D. (2009) Real-life Teaching in a Virtual World, *Campus Technology*, (February), http://campustechnology.com/articles/2009/02/18/real-life-teaching-in-a-virtual-world.aspx.

Hughes, B., Joshi, I. and Wareham, J. (2008) Health 2.0 and Medicine 2.0: tensions and controversies in the field, *Journal of Medical Internet Research*, **10** (3), e23, www.ncbi.nlm.nih.gov/pmc/articles/PMC2553249/.

Issenberg, S. B., McGaghie, W. C., Petrusa, E. R., Lee Gordon, D. and Scalese, R. J. (2005) Features and Uses of High-fidelity Medical Simulations that Lead to Effective Learning: a BEME systematic review, *Medical Teacher*, **27** (1), 10–28.

Jarmon, L., Traphagan, T., Mayrath, M. and Trivedi, A. (2009) Virtual World Teaching, Experiential Learning, and Assessment: an interdisciplinary communication course in Second Life, *Computers and Education*, **53** (1), 169–182.

Johnson, L., Levine, A., Smith, R. and Stone, S. (2010) *The 2010 Horizon Report*, The New Media Consortium, http://wp.nmc.org/horizon2010/.

Kamel Boulos, M. N. and Burden, D. (2007) Web GIS in Practice V: 3-D interactive and real-time mapping in Second Life, *International Journal of Health Geographics*, **6**, 51(16p), www.ij-healthgeographics.com/series/1476-072X-Gis.

Kamel Boulos, M. N. and Toth-Cohen, S. (2008) The University of Plymouth Sexual Health SIM Experience in Second Life: evaluation and reflections after 1 year, *Health Information and Libraries Journal*, **26**, 279–288.

Kamel Boulos, M. N. and Wheeler, S. (2007) The Emerging Web 2.0 Social Software: an enabling suite of sociable technologies in health and health care education, *Health Information and Libraries Journal*, **24**, 2–23.

Kamel Boulos, M. N., Hetherington, L. and Wheeler, S. (2007) Second Life: an overview of the potential of 3-D virtual worlds in medical and health education, *Health Information and Libraries Journal*, **24** (4), 233–45.

Kamel Boulos, M. N., Maramba, I. and Wheeler, S. (2006) Wikis, Blogs and Podcasts: a new generation of web-based tools for virtual collaborative clinical practice and education, *BMC Medical Education*, **6** (41), www.biomedcentral.com/1472-6920/6/41.

Kamel Boulos, M. N., Ramloll, R., Jones, R. and Toth-Cohen, S. (2008) Web 3D for Public, Environmental and Occupational Health: early examples from Second Life, *International Journal of Environmental Research and Public Health*, **5** (4), 290–317.

Kamel Boulos, M. N., Scotch, M., Cheung, K. H. and Burden, D. (2008) Web GIS in Practice VI: a demo 'playlist' of geo-mashups for public health neogeographers, *International Journal of Health Geographics*, **7**, 38–53, www.ij-healthgeographics.com/series/1476-072X-Gis.

Kaphingst, K. A., Persky, S., McCall, C., Lachance, C., Beall, A. C. and Blascovich, J. (2009a) Testing Communication Strategies to Convey Genomic Concepts Using Virtual Reality Technology, *Journal of Health Communication*, **14** (4), 384–99.

Kaphingst, K. A., Persky, S., McCall, C., Lachance, C., Loewenstein, J., Beall, A. C. and Blascovich, J. (2009b) Testing the Effects of Educational Strategies on Comprehension of a Genomic Concept Using Virtual Reality Technology, *Patient Education and Counselling*, **77** (2), 224–30.

Kapp, K. M. and O'Driscoll, T. (2010) *Learning in 3D: adding a new dimension to enterprise learning and collaboration*, Wiley, http://books.google.com/books?id=d6lSyf3HNLIC.

Ketelhut, D. J. and Niemi, S. M. (2007) Emerging Technologies in Education and Training: applications for the laboratory animal science community, *ILAR Journal*, **48** (2), 163–169.

Kinnison, T., Forrest, N. D., Frean, S. P. and Baillie, S. (2009) Teaching Bovine Abdominal Anatomy: use of a haptic simulator, *Anatomical Sciences Education*, **2** (6), 280–285, cover.

Kirkpatrick, M. (2009) Two New Apps Superimpose Wikipedia Over Your iPhone Camera View of the World, *ReadWriteWeb*, (2 October), www.readwriteweb.com/archives/two_apps_now_superimpose_wikipedia_over_your_iphon.php.

Krueger, A., Ludwig, A. and Ludwig, D. (2009) Universal Design for Virtual Worlds, *Journal of Virtual World Research*, **2** (3), http://jvwresearch.org/index.php?_cms=1256151694.

Lafsky, M. (2009) Can Training in Second Life Teach Doctors to Save Real Lives? *Discover Magazine*, (16 July), http://discovermagazine.com/2009/jul-aug/15-can-medical-students-learn-to-save-real-lives-in-second-life.

Lamb, D. (2007) Could Simulated Emergency Procedures Practised in a Static Environment Improve the Clinical Performance of a Critical Care Air Support Team (CCAST)? A literature review, *Intensive Critical Care Nursing*, **23**, 33–42.

Leighton, K. and Dubas, J. (2009) Simulated Death: an innovative approach to teaching end-of-life care, *Clinical Simulation in Nursing*, **5**, e223–230.

Lemley, T. and Burnham, J. F. (2009) Web 2.0 Tools in Medical and Nursing School Curricula, *Journal of the Medical Library Association*, **97** (1), 50-52.

Levy, P., Ford, N., Foster, J., Madden, A., Miller, D., Nunes, M. B., McPherson, M. and Webber, S. (2003) Educational Informatics: an emerging research agenda, *Journal of Information Science*, **29**, 298–310.

Linden, P. (2005) New Residents in Second Life this Fall – Campus: Second Life program continues! *Second Life Forums*, (3 September), http://forums.secondlife.com/showthread.php?t=60133?lang=en.

Lofgren, E. T. and Fefferman, N. H. (2007) The Untapped Potential of Virtual Game Worlds to Shed Light on Real World Epidemics, *Lancet Infectious Diseases*, **7**, 625–629.

Lombardi, M. M. (2007) *Authentic Learning for the 21st Century: an overview* (ELI White Papers, ELI3009), EDUCAUSE Learning Initiative, www.educause.edu/ELI/AuthenticLearningforthe21stCen/156769.

McElhinney, E. (2009) Exploring Nursing Students' Decision-making while in a Second Life Clinical Simulation Laboratory. Dr. Jacqueline McCallum, Val Ness, Theresa Price, Andy Whiteford, *Glasgow Caledonian University, School of Health – Virtual Worlds*, http://caledonianblogs.net/soh-secondlife/2009/09/16/exploring-nursing-students%E2%80%99-decision-making-while-in-a-second-life-clinical-simulation-laboratory-dr-jacqueline-mccallum-val-ness-theresa-price-andy-whiteford/.

McKenzie, F. D., Hubbard, T. W., Ullian, J. A., Garcia, H. M., Castelino, R. J. and Gliva, G. A. (2006) Medical Student Evaluation Using Augmented Standardized Patients: preliminary results, *Studies in Health Technology and Informatics*, **119**, 379–84.

McLean, R., Richards, B.H. and Wardman, J.I. (2007) The Effect of Web 2.0 on the future of medical practice and education: Darwikinian evolution or folksonomic revolution?, *Medical Journal of Australia*, **187**, 174–7.

Mantovani, F., Castelnuovo, G., Gaggioli, A. and Riva, G. (2003) Virtual Reality Training for Health-care Professionals, *CyberPsychology & Behavior*, **6** (4), 389–395.

Maru, D. S. R., Sharma, A., Andrews, J., Basu, S., Thapa, J., Oza, S., Bashyal, C., Acharya, B. and Schwarz, R. (2009) Global Health Delivery 2.0: using open-access technologies for transparency and operations research, *PLoS Medicine*, **6** (12), e1000158.

Mattheos, N., Stefanovic, N., Apse, P., Attstrom, R., Buchanan, J., Brown, P., Camilleri, A., Care, R., Fabrikant, E., Gundersen, S., Honkala, S., Johnson, L., Jonas, I., Kavadella, A., Moreira, J., Peroz, I., Perryer, D. G., Seemann, R., Tansy, M., Thomas, H. F., Tsuruta, J., Uribe, S., Urtane, I., Walsh, T. F., Zimmerman, J. and Walmsley, A. D. (2008) Potential of Information Technology in Dental Education, *European Journal of Dental Education*, **12** (suppl. 1), 85–92.

Mettler, L. L. and Dewan, P. (2009) Virtual Reality Simulators in Gynecological Endoscopy: a surging new wave, *JSLS: Journal of the Society of Laparoendoscopic Surgeons*, **13** (3), 279–86.

Miller, J. (2008) Simulation and Teaching in Second Life. Presented at *Best Practices in Allied Health/Health Sciences*, Renton Technical Community College, (7 May), www.slideshare.net/jsvavoom/games-for-health-conf-baltimore.

Miller, J. (2009) Medical Simulation in the Virtual World of Second Life, (15 March), *MUVErs* (www.muvers.org/), www.youtube.com/watch?v=TkuLAOzL0zU.

Morrison, B., Scarcello, M., Thibeault, L. and Walker, D. (2009) The Use of a Simulated Nursing Practice Lab in a Distance Practical Nursing Program, *Clinical Simulation in Nursing*, **5**, e67–e71.

MUVErsLLC. (2009), http://muversllc.blogspot.com/.

Nehring, W. M. and Lashley, F. R. (2009) Nursing Simulation: a review of the past 40 years, *Simulation and Gaming*, **40** (4), 528–552.

Nelson, D. L. and Blenkin, C. (2007) The Power of Online Role-Play Simulations: technology in nursing education, *International Journal of Nursing Education and Scholarship*, **4** (1), Article 1, www.bepress.com/ijnes/vol4/iss1/art1.

New York University, School of Medicine, Department of Educational Informatics (2009) [*Homepage.*] NYU Medical Center, http://dei.med.nyu.edu/.

Nursing 211 (2007) Second Life Medical Field Trips, September–December, http://nurs211f07.blogspot.com/.

Oddsson, L. I. E., Karlsson, R., Konrad, J., Ince, S., Williams, S. R. and Zemkova, E. (2007) A Rehabilitation Tool for Functional Balance Using Altered Gravity and Virtual Reality, *Journal of NeuroEngineering and Rehabilitation*, **4** (1), 25.

Oleetzel (2008) *Testis Tour on OSU Medicine*,
    www.youtube.com/watch?v=O1YuRSyzBAE.

Paine, H. (2009) College of Nursing Second Life Public Health Office, *SLHealthy*,
    (13 October),
    http://slhealthy.wetpaint.com/page/College+of+Nursing+Second+Life+Public
    +Health+Office.

Pentland, A., Lazer, D., Brewer, D. and Heibeck, T. (2009) Using Reality Mining to
    Improve Public Health and Medicine, *Studies in Health Technology and Informatics*,
    149, 93–102.

Phillips, J. and Berge, Z. L. (2009) Second Life for Dental Education, *Journal of Dental
    Education*, **73** (11), 1260–4.

Raeside, W. (2008) Medics Enter Virtual World, *Reporter*, **190**, 11,
    www3.imperial.ac.uk/pls/portallive/docs/1/40465710.PDF.

Ramloll, R., Beedasy, J., Stamm, B. H., Piland, M., Cunningham, B., Kirkwood, A.,
    Massad, P., Spearman, R., Patel, A., Tivis, R. and Kelchner, C. (2006) Distance
    Learning and Simulation Technologies to Support Bioterrorism Preparedness
    Education, *Proceedings of the ISCA 21st International Conference*, 235–41,
    www.isu.edu/irh/IBAPP/documents/ramesh_IRH_submission_CATA%202006
    %20S102.pdf.

Reger, G. M. and Gahm, G. A. (2008) Virtual Reality Exposure Therapy for Active
    Duty Soldiers, *Journal of Clinical Psychology*, **64** (8), 940–6.

Reger, G. M., Gahm, G. A., Rizzo, A. A., Swanson, R. and Duma, S. (2009) Soldier
    Evaluation of the Virtual Reality Iraq, *Telemedicine and e-Health*, **15** (1), 101–4.

Reiner, B. and Siegel, E. (2008) The Potential for Gaming Techniques in Radiology
    Education and Practice, *Journal of the American College of Radiology*, **5** (2), 110–14.

Rizzo, A. A., Difede, J., Rothbaum, B. O., Johnston, S., McLay, R. N., Reger, G.,
    Gahm, G., Parsons, T., Graap, K. and Pair, J. (2009) VR PTSD Exposure
    Therapy Results with Active Duty OIF/OEF Combatants, *Studies in Health
    Technology and Informatics*, **142**, 277–82.

Rizzo, A. A., Graap, K., Perlman, K., McLay, R. N., Rothbaum, B. O., Reger, G.,
    Parsons, T., Difede, J. and Pair, J. (2008) Virtual Iraq: initial results from a VR
    exposure therapy application for combat-related PTSD, *Studies in Health Technology
    and Informatics*, **132**, 420–5.

Rizzo, A., Pair, J., McNerney, P. J., Eastlund, E., Manson, B., Gratch, J., Hill, R. and
    Swartout, B. (2005) Development of a VR Therapy Application for Iraq War
    Military Personnel with PTSD, *Studies in Health Technology and Informatics*, **111**, 407–
    13.

Rosen, K. R. (2008) The History of Medical Simulation, *Journal of Critical Care*, **23**
    (2), 157–66.

Rothbaum, B. O., Hodges, L. F., Ready, D., Graap, K. and Alarcon, R. D. (2001)
    Virtual Reality Exposure Therapy for Vietnam Veterans with Posttraumatic
    Stress Disorder, *Journal of Clinical Psychiatry*, **62** (8), 617–22.

Royse, M. A. and Newton, S. E. (2007) How Gaming is Used as an Innovative Strategy for Nursing Education, *Nursing Education Perspectives*, **28** (5), 263–7.

Russomano, T., Cardoso, R. B., Fernandes, J., Cardoso, P. G., Alves, J. M., Pianta, C. D., Souza, H. P. and Lopes, M. H. (2009) Tele-surgery: a new virtual tool for medical education, *Studies in Health Technology and Informatics*, **150**, 866–70.

Schmidt, B. and Stewart, S. (2009) Implementing the Virtual Reality Learning Environment: Second Life, *Nurse Education*, **34** (4), 152–5.

Schreiber, W. E. and Giustini, D. M. (2009) Pathology in the Era of Web 2.0, *American Journal of Clinical Pathology*, **132**, 824–828.

Skiba, D. J. (2009) Emerging Technologies Center: Nursing Education 2.0: a second look at Second Life, *Nursing Education Perspectives*, **30** (2), 129–31, http://nln.allenpress.com/nlnonline/?request=get-document&issn=1536-5026&volume=030&issue=02&page=0129.

Skiba, D. J., Connors, H. R. and Jeffries, P. R. (2008) Information Technologies and the Transformation of Nursing Education, *Nursing Outlook*, **56** (5), 225–30.

SLHealthy (2007–), http://slhealthy.wetpaint.com/.

Smith, C. E. (2009) Developing Simulation Scenarios for Perioperative Nursing Core Competencies and Patient Safety, *Perioperative Nursing Clinics*, **4** (2), 157–165.

Snyder, C. W., Vandromme, M. J., Tyra, S. L. and Hawn, M. T. (2009) Proficiency-based Laparoscopic and Endoscopic Training with Virtual Reality Simulators: a comparison of proctored and independent approaches, *Journal of Surgical Education*, **66** (4), 201–7.

Spallek, H., O'Donnell, J., Clayton, M., Anderson, P. and Krueger, A. (2010) Paradigm Shift or Annoying Distraction – Emerging Implications of Web 2.0 for Clinical Practice, *Applied Clinical Informatics*, **1** (2), 96–115, www.schattauer.de/de/magazine/uebersicht/zeitschriften-a-z/applied-clinical-informatics/contents/archive/issue/1062/manuscript/12955.html.

Stephens, M. R. (2009) *Exploring Virtual Worlds as a Platform for Education: the virtual first responder*, www.slideshare.net/marqueA2/final-sl-for-ed-vfr-03june2009.

Stewart, S., Pope, D. and Duncan, D. (2009) Using Second Life to Enhance ACCEL an Online Accelerated Nursing BSN Program, *Studies in Health Technology and Informatics*, **146**, 636–40.

Strangman, N. and Hall, T. (2003) *Virtual Reality/Computer Simulations*, National Center on Accessing the General Curriculum, www.cast.org/publications/ncac/ncac_vr.html.

Susi, T., Johannesson, M. and Backlund, P. (2007) *Serious Games – An Overview*, (Technical Report HS- IKI -TR-07-001), Interreg IIIC Programme, DISTRICT (Developing Industrial Strategies Through Innovative Cluster and Technologies), Serious Games Cluster and Business Network (SER3VG), University of Skövde, School of Humanities and Informatics, www.sysope.fr/content/download/523/2932/file/Serious%20Games_an%20overview.pdf.

Svoboda, E. and Richards, B. (2009) Compensating for Anterograde Amnesia: a new training method that capitalizes on emerging smartphone technologies, *Journal of the International Neuropsychology Society*, **15** (4), 629–38.

Telner, D., Chan, D., Chester, B., Marlow, B., Meuser, J., Arthur Rothman, A. and Harvey, B. (2010) Game-based versus Traditional Case-based Learning: comparing effectiveness in stroke continuing medical education, *Canadian Family Physician*, September, **56** (9), e345–e51, www.cfp.ca/cgi/content/abstract/56/9/e345.

Trelease, R. B. (2008) Diffusion of Innovations: smartphones and wireless anatomy learning resources, *Anatomical Sciences Education*, **1** (6), 233–9.

USC Institute for Creative Technologies (homepage), http://ict.usc.edu/.

Vance, K., Howe, W. and Dellavalle, R. P. (2009) Social Internet Sites as a Source of Public Health Information, *Dermatologic Clinics*, **27**, 133–136.

Versel, N. (2009) Mobile Video Systems Link ED with Ambulances to Jump-start Triage, *Hospitals and Health Networks*, **83** (5), 12.

Virtually Better (2009) www.virtuallybetter.com/.

Walker, C., Miller, J., Merrick, S., Holmes, P., Peng, B., Goodman, J., Crawford, C., Taylor, K. and Tevlin, T. (2009) Medical Roleplays in Second Life, a Virtual World, *MUVErsLLC*, (1 December), http://muversllc.blogspot.com/2009/12/medical-roleplays-in-second-life.html.

Walker, V. L. (2009) *Using 3D Virtual Environments in Counselor Education for Mental Health Interviewing and Diagnosis: student perceived learning benefits*. Dissertation, Regent University, Virginia, United States. ProQuest Publication #AAT3374779. April, www.scribd.com/doc/23663272/Victoria-L-Walker-Dissertation ; www.regent.edu/acad/schedu/pdfs/abstracts/walker_2009.pdf.

Weiner, E. E. (2008) Technology: the interface to nursing educational informatics, Preface, *Nursing Clinics of North America*, **43** (4), ix–x.

Weiner, E. E. and Tragenstein, P. A. (2009) The Emerging Role of Educational Informatics, *Studies in Health Technology and Informatics*, **146**, 567–71.

Wick, M. R. (2009) Reflections on Pathology and 'Web 2.0', *American Journal of Clinical Pathology*, **132**, 813–815.

Wiecha, J., Heyden, R., Sternthal, E. and Merialdi, M. (2010) Learning in a Virtual World: experience with using Second Life for medical education, *Journal of Medical Internet Research*, **12** (1), e1, www.jmir.org/2010/1/e1/.

Wong, L. (2009) UW-Green Bay Second Life Nursing Complex, *LTDC Online News*, (6 May), http://blogs.uww.edu/ltdc/uw-green-bay-second-life-nursing-complex/.

Wood, D. P., Webb-Murphy, J., Center, K., McLay, R., Koffman, R., Johnston, S., Spira, J., Pyne, J. M. and Wiederhold, B. K. (2009) Combat-related Post-traumatic Stress Disorder: a case report using virtual reality graded exposure therapy with physiological monitoring with a female Seabee, *Military Medicine*, **174** (11), 1215–22.

Yellowlees, P. M. and Cook, J. N. (2006) Education about Hallucinations Using an Internet Virtual Reality System: a qualitative survey, *Academic Psychiatry*, **30** (6), 534–539.

Zielke, M. A., Roome, T. C. and Krueger, A. B. (2009) A Composite Adult Learning Model for Virtual World Residents with Disabilities: a case study of the virtual ability Second Life island, *Journal of Virtual Worlds Research*, **2** (1), [1–21], http://journals.tdl.org/jvwr/article/view/417/461.

CHAPTER 4

Supporting learners via Web 2.0

Laura Cobus-Kuo

Introduction

Public health professionals are responsible for using various forms of media (TV, radio, newspapers, research, the web) to communicate with the public. Use of newer Web 2.0 tools where content can be added, edited or revised, sometimes by many authors, arguably increases the risk of potentially biased or harmful health information. It therefore becomes the public health professional's responsibility to learn the skills needed to critically appraise web content that hasn't gone through the traditional peer-review process. It is important for health professionals and educators to become active participants and contributors to Web 2.0 systems and, moreover, to assist in developing a system and infrastructure that supports educators in successfully incorporating technology into the classroom. This chapter addresses these issues, in particular the use of blogs and wikis in healthcare education.

Web 2.0 in higher education

Higher education is in the midst of a major transformation as it tries to keep up with the impact that new technologies such as Web 2.0 are having upon it. Universities are only at the early stages of coming to terms with the changes technology is creating; however, the expectation from students is that technology will play a major role in their education (Finkelman and Kenner, 2009) – and they're ready for it (Collis and Moonen, 2008)! Institutions of higher education must ensure that educators are on the front line of this ever-changing landscape and have the skills to successfully incorporate information technology into the curriculum.

In the health sciences there have been calls for a systematic revision of the education of healthcare professionals by embedding technology and information-seeking skills into the curriculum (Association of American Medical Colleges, 1998a; Association of American Medical Colleges, 1998b; Association of College and Research Libraries, 2000; Finkelman and Kenner, 2009; Institute of Medicine, 2003; Medical Library Association, 2007; National League for Nursing, 2008; Yasnoff et al., 2001). The health sciences have become an 'information-processing enterprise' (Shaw, 2010), reinforcing the need for health professionals to have proficient information technology and information gathering skills.

At present, there is little in the literature systematically reviewing and assessing the use of Web 2.0 in the classroom (Luo, 2010; Skiba and Barton, 2009). At best, it is only 'slowly' being incorporated into health and medically related curricula (Kamel Boulos and Wheeler, 2007; Lemley and Burnham, 2009). As a way to address the demand for revision of healthcare education so as to better meet the changing needs of students, a medical librarian developed and delivered a graduate course for a Master's in Public Health programme that incorporated Web 2.0 technologies into the curriculum. The idea of the course was a direct result of several meetings with the library and the School of Public Health that focused on ways to improve research skills and, ultimately, the curriculum.

Blogs and wikis, two of the many types of Web 2.0 technologies, were the tools used to formally assess students in the course. Blogs and wikis, in particular, have been shown to be of great use in higher education (Collis and Moonen, 2008) both in inciting active collaboration and as being valuable in group work. Blogs (short for weblogs) are 21st-century diaries. The web-based narrative chronicles the many ideas of an author or authors over time, the entries being published in reverse chronological order, with the most recent entry listed first.

Blogs and wikis

Blogs are reflective in nature and can vary in length from post to post. They allow comments from readers, whether in an open or password-protected environment, thus encouraging the participatory engagement that defines Web 2.0. Blogs not only include written text, but can also include images, video and audio files, along with links to other websites. Most blogging software provides Really Simple Syndication (RSS) capability for instant subscription. RSS is an XML tool that pushes content to a user, based on their personal subscription settings. In other words, a user can 'subscribe' to a blog, newspaper, journal table of contents, etc. and be notified the instant it is updated. The information is fed to the user via their preferred method, such as e-mail, browser updates or a web-based aggregator. Blogging software is free or available at a minimal cost and, like most Web 2.0 tools, is very easy to use. It can be available as an online open-source application or as a downloadable and installed application that enables the user to blog using desktop software (Wikipedia, 2010a).

Blogging in the health sciences is an accepted mode of communicating medical research (Holmes and Dubinsky, 2009) and is embraced by both health consumers and healthcare professionals. Research shows that 33% of all internet users read blogs regularly and that 12% admit to being bloggers at some point in their life (Smith, 2008). Data also suggest that 16% of all blogs are focused on health-related topics, whereas science accounts for 19% of all blogs (Sussman, 2009). Assuming that there is overlap between the categories of health and science, this could account for over one-third of all blogs in existence.

Wikis are collaborative, web-based tools that sometimes allow many authors to edit and add content based on their own expertise on a given topic. A wiki can be as short as a one-page document, but it has the potential to become infinitely large. Wikipedia is the best known wiki, with over 3 million pages in English (Wikipedia, 2010b), and has been shown to be as accurate as, arguably, the best known print encyclopedia, *Encyclopaedia Britannica* (Giles, 2005). Just as with blogs, wikis are easy to use and can include text, video, audio and images. They can be either open or closed, meaning that anyone can read and edit an open wiki or only those with authorized passwords can edit the 'closed' site. Wikis encourage active participation by the community and rely upon the peer-review process of constant edits, changes and updates. The continual regulation provided by the community leads to a 'darwikinism' (McLean, Richards and Wardman, 2007) or evolution of good-quality information that removes vandalism or inaccurate information. Moreover, authors will often refer to authoritative resources that justify their contributions or revisions (Cain and Fox, 2009).

In the health sciences, wikis can be used for a variety of purposes, including but not limited to institutional repositories, organizational procedures or policy manuals, data collection, group projects, journal or book clubs, grand rounds, collaboratively written articles or books, and emergency response tools (Chimato, 2007; Grassley and Bartoletti, 2009; Holmes and Dubinsky, 2009). Blogger and medical librarian David Rothman maintains an ever-growing list of medical wikis ranging in topics from AIDS to medical billing to surgery (Rothman, 2010). Wikis are challenging and changing the traditional model of publishing by offering a platform of constant renewal and currency.

Critical appraisal and Web 2.0

Critical appraisal of information has always been a hallmark of higher education, but with newer Web 2.0 self-publishing tools, health students need to be more rigid in their critical assessment strategies towards and analysis of information that has not been vetted by a review board (McGee and Begg, 2008). Students must learn how to think about potential bias and limitations when engaging with Web 2.0 resources, by comprehending the difference between quality information and poor information (Cain and Fox, 2009; McGee and Begg, 2008). Web 2.0 provides an opportunity for both educators and learners to understand the benefits and shortcomings of Web 2.0 applications by training students how to use the technology effectively, efficiently and ethically (Hughes et al., 2009). Future healthcare professionals will not only be responsible for knowing how to navigate in a constantly changing technological environment, but they will also be responsible for teaching colleagues and consumers how to use information technologies (Brixey and Warren, 2009).

Among many possible barriers to incorporating Web 2.0 and other digital information technology tools into the curriculum are: inadequately trained faculty (Griffin-Sobel et al., 2010; Jeffries, 2008; Yasnoff et al., 2001), and the fact that technologies are not known, not valued, perceived as too difficult to implement or seen as a 'solution in search of a problem' (Collis and Moonen, 2008). One way to address such barriers and to implement technology into the curriculum is to develop partnerships with librarians and libraries (Cobus, 2008; Cohen, 2008; Griffin-Sobel et al., 2010; Lemley and Burnham, 2009; Phillips and Bonsteel, 201).

Medical librarians are early adopters of technology on university campuses. They have also been long-time advocates of information literacy (IL) or the 'ability to know when information is needed, [and] to be able to locate, evaluate, and effectively use that information for lifelong learning and problem solving' (American Library Association, 1989). To educate students and future healthcare professionals to become conversant with IL skills and information technology, librarians use 'active learning' strategies in the classroom. Active learning requires students to actively engage with, debate and deconstruct information in a collaborative manner (Bonwell and Eison, 1991; Gradowski, Snavely and Dempsey, 1998). Such learning is often in the form of hands-on computer and IL exercises, used as a way to engage students in the learning process and to develop critical thinking skills (Association of College and Research Libraries, 2003). Active learning requires careful planning by the teacher and structured exercises to ensure that students connect with the learning process, regardless of learning styles. Furthermore, active learning increases student learning (Gradowski, Snavely and Dempsey, 1998). Thus, it should come as no surprise that medical librarians would be interested in incorporating Web 2.0 technologies into the IL curriculum and use active learning strategies as a way to enhance learning (Cobus, 2009; Lemley and Burnham, 2009). Web 2.0 in IL is an opportunity to adjust pedagogical styles and incorporate active learning that includes interactive web-based resources that are user-driven and collaborative (Godwin, 2009).

Case study: Information research in public health at Hunter College

Hunter College is part of the largest and most diverse urban public university system in the United States, the City University of New York (CUNY). Students pursue degrees in both undergraduate and graduate programmes. The Department of Urban Public Health (UPH) prepares its students 'to promote health and prevent disease among residents of urban communities' (Hunter College Department of Urban Public Health, 2010). The Health Professions Library supports the curricular and research needs of UPH students and faculty. *Information Research in Public Health, PH 770* was a graduate-level elective that was developed and delivered by a librarian for the UPH programme. The librarian incorporated Web 2.0 technology as the primary mode of assessment; specifically, blogs and wikis were used to evaluate IL skills, collaboration and group work, research skills and communication skills.

Course description

The course was described in the syllabus as follows:

> This course provides the opportunity for students to pursue the theoretical and practical principles of information research in public health. This course will examine the nature, production and uses of information and the latest developments in information technology and its impact on the public's health. Students will learn the necessary skills to become expert searchers and develop proficiencies in identifying, retrieving, evaluating, and using relevant print, electronic and Internet sources to locate health-based government, evidence based, community, political, and statistical information for in-depth public health research.

The course goals, as stated in the syllabus were:

- Develop effective information-seeking patterns and search strategies focused on public health outcomes.
- Search scholarly databases, government resources, search engines and other electronic information retrieval systems using Boolean and non-Boolean strategies.
- Apply the use of databases, spreadsheets, search engines, and other internet resources to public health research practices.
- Evaluate, assess and appraise information/database quality.
- Demonstrate and understand digital media's relevance to public health.

The course was delivered during the summer over a 6-week period, with lectures being held for three hours two times per week. Initially there were ten students enrolled in the course, with one student withdrawing mid-semester. The lectures were held in the library's instructional computer classroom, equipped with 30 computers, allowing each student to have their own PC. The instructor's computer was situated at the front of the classroom and had LanSchool, a classroom control system, installed as a means of monitoring student activity on the computers. The course used Blackboard, a web-based classroom management system, to administer all course materials.

Each lecture throughout the semester was skills-based and built upon the overriding course goals of developing search and research strategies in the field of public health. Each lecture included active learning exercises applied to the various research tools so as to ensure that the research principles were understood. For example, the first lecture started with a discussion of the history of publishing, all within the context of public health. The lecture moved from clay tablets to papyrus to the printing press and ended with Web 2.0 technology. At the end of the first lecture, the instructor demonstrated the blog and wiki utility in Blackboard and created an in-class active-learning exercise in order for the students to familiarize themselves with the new technology.

To learn critical assessment of both scholarly and non-peer-reviewed sources of information, the students were required to use the criteria developed by the Johns Hopkins Sheridan Libraries, which include authorship, publishing body, point of view or bias, referral to other sources, verifiability, currency, how to distinguish propaganda, misinformation and disinformation, and the mechanics of determining authorship, publishing body, and currency on the internet (Kirk, 1996). Students were required to understand the difference between primary and secondary sources, the virtues of evidence-based authoritative information and the pitfalls of poor information.

Within Blackboard, the home page was set up as a course blog. The course blog was not graded, but was recommended as the primary mode of communication between students and between teacher and students. It was considered an informal virtual place for students to learn the basics of online participatory engagement. The instructor contributed to the blog daily by posting course-related information as a means of teaching blogging etiquette and style. Students followed the teacher's lead and started to add content as posts and comments.

To assess learning, students were required to create weekly individual blogs describing a current event in public health and to create a public health wiki. All assignments were completed within the course management tool, Blackboard. Although Blackboard is not as 'authentic' as other blogging and wiki utilities, being open only to those enrolled in the course for the duration of the semester, it did allow for easy assessment within a controlled environment, as the instructor could monitor precise online activity for each student in the course. The weekly individual blogging and wiki projects each counted 40% towards the final course grade. The remaining 20% was based on attendance and in-class participation.

Blog assignment

Each student in PH 770 was given a blog space in Blackboard, set up by the instructor. Students were required to post on their blogs two times per week on a current public health issue and to comment on at least two other blogs by each posting deadline (Figure 4.1). To frame the assignment, there were three overarching goals that the students were to follow. The first goal, information retrieval, required students to find at least four authoritative online sources relevant to a particular public health current event. The second goal, self-publishing, was completed through a reflective journal entry of between 250 and 350 words that seamlessly incorporated hyperlinks to the four different sources. Participation was the third goal, which was accomplished through making thoughtful comments on the blogs of other students. To evaluate the blogs, a grading rubric was developed that was also available to the students.

The rubric was provided as a guideline to assess the students' ability to find and incorporate authoritative online resources and to write a thoughtful piece within the specified guidelines, all while using the blogging technology correctly (e.g. creating active hyperlinks). As the semester progressed, there was a marked improvement with the students' ability to hit the right register expected in blogs, while following the appropriate blogging etiquette. But more importantly, over time the students mastered

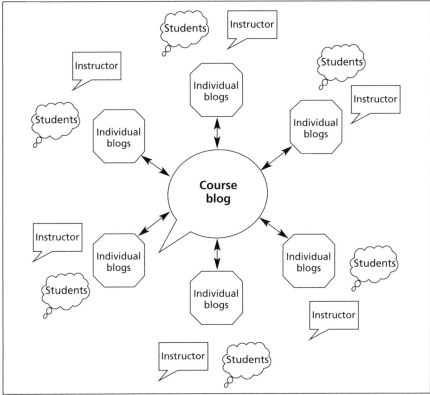

Figure 4.1 *The various models of blogging used in the course*
Note: The course blog was not graded and was the primary mode of
communication between everyone in the course. The individual blogs were
graded and required participation through commenting as a means of
further engagement of the learning process.

the process of identifying what are considered to be authoritative sources, as opposed
to questionable or biased sources.

Wiki assignment

The wiki assignment was an online and interactive annotated bibliography (Engstrom
and Jewett, 2005). The scope of the wiki matched the subject tracks of the UPH
programme: community health education, nutrition, and environmental and occupational
health. The intended audience of the wiki was public health students and professionals,
as opposed to health consumers. The instructor used a grading rubric to evaluate the
wiki and this was used as a guideline to assess the students' mastery of critically assessing
online information, creating a logical structure and writing exemplary annotations.

Five goals framed the wiki assignment. The first goal was to find three types of
authoritative information: government, non-government and research articles. The next

goal was to design a well organized wiki. The third was to annotate each resource succinctly using 150 words or fewer. The annotation was to be descriptive, summative, reflective and critical. The students were also to provide evaluative information on the author's credentials, the intended audience and the article's usefulness within the scope of the overall bibliography. The fourth goal, critical appraisal, was tied into the overall course through class lectures, discussions and the Johns Hopkins guidelines (Kirk, 1996). Public discourse, where learners presented a thoughtful oral presentation and discussion of the wiki experience to the class as a whole, framed the fifth goal.

The wiki assignment was divided into two phases (Figure 4.2). During the first phase, over a 3-week period, students were required to focus on one of the three UPH subject tracks: nutrition, community health education or environmental and occupational health. The students were grouped into three teams, each team having three students and one member from one of the three subject tracks. The teams were given a wiki space on Blackboard and worked within a closed-team environment. The learners were required to find and annotate resources on their subject areas and encouraged to focus on an area of interest. They were required to find and annotate between four and eight US Government web-based tools, non-government web-based tools and evidence-based research articles discussing their subject that had been published within the last five years.

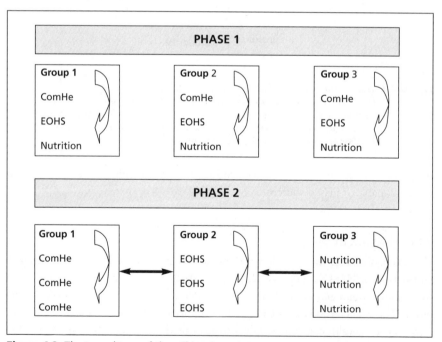

Figure 4.2 *The two phases of the wiki assignment*
Note: In the first phase the students worked within a closed wiki environment based on their subject, whereas the second phase was an open wiki where the groups could view the wiki pages and edit within their own subject group.

During the second phase of the assignment, the students worked within an open wiki environment where all were able to see and review the wiki pages. However, during this second phase the students were required to work within their subject-specific teams: all of the nutrition students worked together, as did the environmental and occupational health students and community health education students. The subject groups were required to collaborate and select the top six to ten resources out of the possible 12 to 24 resources discovered during the first, individual half of the assignment and to provide a table of contents with a logical organizational structure. On the last day of the class, the subject groups presented their sections of the wiki. They were required to provide a detailed account describing the criteria used in deciding which government and non-government sources to include and exclude, based on the Johns Hopkins guidelines, their reasoning in selecting the best evidence-based research articles, the challenges encountered and the collaborative roles and responsibilities within their team.

Lessons learned

To successfully implement Web 2.0 technologies as assessment tools, the instructor met and worked with the University's Technology Teaching and Learning Group (TTLG) during the initial brainstorming phase of course development. TTLG's mission is to support faculty with their educational endeavour of thoughtfully incorporating technology into the curriculum. Its support was invaluable and key to the success of the course, as it helped the instructor fulfil the course goals and pedagogical objectives, while also providing assistance in learning the blog and wiki utilities in Blackboard. The class size of nine students also contributed to the overall course success. For example, a lot of time was spent not only reading and editing content, but also manually checking the functionality of countless hyperlinks and assessing the authority of the numerous sources embedded in the blogs and wikis. With a larger class size, it would have been necessary to have a Teacher's Assistant (TA) to help with grading assignments and to provide assistance with the technology. The biggest challenge was the varying degrees of computer, technology and research skill of the students. For example, a couple of students were novice internet, e-mail, and word-processing users, as they were 'mature' students with minimal computer experience returning to school, whereas one student was already an avid blogger and another student was a former web-designer. It was therefore extremely helpful to be able to teach in the library's computer classroom, where each student had access to a computer, enabling the instructor to spend time with students who required extra assistance.

Although the students were not formally surveyed or assessed, there was an improvement throughout the semester in their information-seeking skills and ability to critically assess information. They demonstrated a theoretical and practical understanding of the information environment, both print and digital, all within the realm of public health. During the final presentations the students voiced a sense of confidence and excitement at having learned about Web 2.0 technology and the opportunities provided by it.

Recommendations

It is recommended that in the future this course be offered during a traditional fall or spring semester. Teaching during a summer semester provided too short a time and was rushed, given the complexities and newness of the Web 2.0 tools. It would also be prudent to provide examples of expected deliverables early in the semester, in order to allay student anxiety. Using Blackboard was advantageous in terms of being able to closely monitor the students' activity, but it is not an authentic Web 2.0 application. For example, at Hunter College, Blackboard is only available to students during the course and is deactivated once the semester is finished. It would be useful to ensure that the wiki and blogs were made available for future use, whether in Blackboard or on other blog and wiki platforms.

Having the blog and wiki each count for 40% of the overall course grade provided a substantial incentive for the students to take their assignments seriously. However, there is little evidence in the literature that details the success of using these technologies in the classroom. It is thus recommended that qualitative and quantitative assessment of the teaching and learning methods be conducted. Providing podcasts and vodcasts of the lectures, along with having a place for the students to receive ongoing support in creating and delivering Web 2.0 content and design, is also recommended. The final challenge and recommendation is in the expansion and refinement of the Web 2.0 technologies in health sciences curricula. As Web 2.0 technologies change, so should the course content. For example, expanding the blogging assignment to include 'micro-blogging' using Twitter or other newer and popular technologies should be considered. It is also recommended to include design and formatting standards for the various Web 2.0 technologies as the (visual) presentation of information is crucial in effectively engaging a potentially infinite audience. As a way to further refine the comprehension of Web 2.0 technologies, it is recommended that the instructor engage with the students using the technology whenever possible. As the assignments for this course were entirely online, it would be feasible for the instructor to provide online feedback on the individual and group assignments. The instructor's online assessment would reinforce the notion of reflection and collaboration that is essential to Web 2.0 technologies.

References

American Library Association (1989) *Presidential Committee on Information Literacy*, American Library Association.

Association of American Medical Colleges (1998a) *Learning Objectives for Medical School Education: guidelines for medical schools*, https://services.aamc.org/publications/

index.cfm?fuseaction=Product.displayForm&prd_id=198&prv_id=239.

Association of American Medical Colleges (1998b) *Report II: Contemporary Issues in Medicine: medical informatics and population health*, https://services.aamc.org/publications/index.cfm?fuseaction=Product.displayForm&prd_id=199&prv_id=240.

Association of College and Research Libraries (2000) *Information Literacy Competency Standards for Higher Education as a Guideline for Educators*, www.ala.org/ala/mgrps/divs/acrl/standards/informationliteracycompetency.cfm.

Association of College and Research Libraries (2003) *Guidelines for Instruction Programs in Academic Libraries*, www.ala.org/ala/mgrps/divs/acrl/standards/guidelinesinstruction.cfm.

Bonwell, C. C. and Eison, J. A. (1991) *Active Learning: creating excitement in the classroom*, Jossey-Bass.

Brixey, J. J. and Warren, J. J. (2009) Creating Experiential Learning Activities Using Web 2.0 Tools and Technologies: a case study, *Studies in Health Technology and Informatics*, **146**, 613–17.

Cain, J. and Fox, B. I. (2009) Web 2.0 and Pharmacy Education, *American Journal of Pharmaceutical Education*, **73** (7), www.ncbi.nlm.nih.gov/pmc/articles/PMC2779632/pdf/ajpe120.pdf.

Chimato, M. C. (2007) It's a Wiki Wiki World, *Medical Reference Services Quarterly*, **26**, 169–90.

Cobus, L. (2008) Integrating Information Literacy into the Education of Public Health Professionals: roles for librarians and the library, *Journal of the Medical Library Association*, **96** (1), 28–33.

Cobus, L. (2009) Using Blogs and Wikis in a Graduate Public Health Course, *Medical Reference Services Quarterly*, **28** (1), 22–32.

Cohen, S. F. (2008) Taking 2.0 to the Faculty, *College and Research Libraries News*, **69** (8), 472–5.

Collis, B. and Moonen, J. (2008) Web 2.0 Tools and Processes in Higher Education: quality perspectives, *Educational Media International*, **45** (2), 93–106.

Engstrom, M. E. and Jewett, D. (2005) Collaborative Learning the Wiki Way, *TechTrends: Linking Research and Practice to Improve Learning*, **49** (6), 12.

Finkelman, A. W., Kenner, C. and American Nurses Association (2009) *Teaching IOM: implications of the Institute of Medicine reports for nursing education* (2nd edn), American Nurses Association.

Giles, J. (2005) Special Report: internet encyclopaedias go head to head, *Nature*, **438**, 900.

Godwin, P. (2009) Information Literacy and Web 2.0: is it just hype? *Program: Electronic Library and Information Systems*, **43** (3), 264–74.

Gradowski, G., Snavely, L., Dempsey, P. and Association of College and Research Libraries, Instruction Section, Teaching Methods Committee (1998) *Designs for Active Learning: a sourcebook of classroom strategies for information education*, Association of College and Research Libraries.

Grassley, J. S. and Bartoletti, R. (2009) Wikis and Blogs: tools for online interaction. *Nurse Educator*, **34** (5), 209–13.

Griffin-Sobel, J., Acee, A., Sharoff, L., Cobus-Kuo, L., Woodstock-Wallace, A. and
     Dornbaum, M. (2010) A Transdisciplinary Approach to Faculty Development in
     Nursing Education Technology, *Nursing Education Perspectives*, **31** (1), 41–3.
Holmes, K. L. and Dubinsky, E. K. (2009) Integration of Web 2.0 Technologies in
     the Translational Research Environment, *Medical Reference Services Quarterly*, **28** (4),
     309–35.
Hughes, B., Joshi, I., Lemonde, H. and Wareham, J. (2009) Junior Physician's Use of
     Web 2.0 for Information Seeking and Medical Education: a qualitative study,
     International Journal of Medical Informatics, **78** (10), 645–55.
Hunter College Department of Urban Public Health (2010) *Program in Urban Public
     Health*, www.hunter.cuny.edu/uph.
Institute of Medicine (2003) *Who Will Keep the Public Healthy?: educating public health
     professionals for the 21st century*, National Academies Press.
Jeffries, P. R. (2008) Getting in S.T.E.P. with Simulations: simulations take educator
     preparation, *Nursing Education Perspectives*, **29** (2), 70–3.
Kamel Boulos, M. N. and Wheeler, S. (2007) The Emerging Web 2.0 Social Software:
     an enabling suite of sociable technologies in health and health care education,
     Health Information and Libraries Journal, **24** (1), 2–23.
Kirk, E. (1996) *Evaluating Internet Information*,
     www.library.jhu.edu.proxy.wexler.hunter.cuny.edu/researchhelp/general/evaluating/.
Lemley, T. and Burnham, J. F. (2009) Web 2.0 Tools in Medical and Nursing School
     Curricula, *Journal of the Medical Library Association*, **97** (1), 49–51.
Luo, L. (2010) Web 2.0 Integration in Information Literacy Instruction: an overview,
     Journal of Academic Librarianship, **36** (1), 32–40.
McGee, J. B. and Begg, M. (2008) What Medical Educators Need to Know About
     Web 2.0, *Medical Teacher*, **30** (2), 164–9.
McLean, R., Richards, B. H. and Wardman, J. I. (2007) The Effect of Web 2.0 on the
     Future of Medical Practice and Education: darwikinian evolution or folksonomic
     revolution, *The Medical Journal of Australia*, **187** (3), 174–7.
Medical Library Association (2007) *Health Information Literacy Task Force*,
     www.mlanet.org/resources/healthlit/tfhil_info.html.
National League for Nursing (2008) *Preparing the Next Generation of Nurses to Practice in
     a Technology-Rich Environment: an informatics agenda*,
     www.nln.org/aboutnln/PositionStatements/.
Phillips, R. M. and Bonsteel, S. H. (2010) The Faculty and Information Specialist
     Partnership: stimulating student interest and experiential learning, *Nurse Educator*,
     35 (3), 136–38.
Rothman, D. (2010) *List of Medical Wikis*, http://davidrothman.net/list-of-medical-wikis/
Shaw, J. (2010) Gutenberg 2.0: Harvard's libraries deal with disruptive change,
     Harvard Magazine, (May–June),
     http://harvardmagazine.com/2010/05/gutenberg-2-0.
Skiba, D. J. and Barton, A. J. (2009) Using Social Software to Transform Informatics

Education, *Studies in Health Technology and Informatics*, **146**, 608–12.

Smith, A. (2008) *New Numbers for Blogging and Blog Readership*, www.pewinternet.org/ Commentary/2008/July/New-numbers-for-blogging-and-blog-readership.aspx.

Sussman, M. (2009) *Day 2: the what and why of blogging – SOTB 2009*, http://technorati.com/blogging/article/day-2-the-what-and-why2/.

Wikipedia (2010a) *Blog Software*, http://en.wikipedia.org/wiki/Blog_software.

Wikipedia (2010b) *Wikipedia: size of Wikipedia*, http://en.wikipedia.org/wiki/Wikipedia:Size_of_Wikipedia.

Yasnoff, W. A., Overhage, J. M., Humphreys, B. L., LaVenture, M., Goodman, K. W., Gatewood, L., Ross, D. A., Reid, J., Hammond, W. E., Dwyer, D., Huff, S. M., Gotham, I., Kukafka, R., Loonsk, J. W. and Wagner, M. M. (2001) A National Agenda for Public Health Informatics, *Journal of Public Health Management and Practice: JPHMP*, **7** (6), 1–21.

CHAPTER 5

Supporting research

Chris Mavergames

Introduction

The online research environment has changed somewhat dramatically over the decade 2000–10, and researchers are now more connected than ever before both to their fellow researchers and to an unprecedented amount of information. It is now possible to 'watch' research as it happens – and in some cases to participate in its development – as one can follow the blogs of well known researchers, receive RSS updates from websites with a research focus, subscribe to podcasts, participate in the creation of wikis and in other collaborative environments, share citations and other bookmarks and join social networks around topic-specific research interests. All of these activities fall under the heading of the so-called Web 2.0, a suite of tools and technologies that has changed the way we interact with and use the web. In an early article on Web 2.0 and medicine, Giustini notes that 'the more we use, share, and exchange information on the web in a continual loop of analysis and refinement, the more open and creative the platform becomes, hence, the more useful it is in our work' (Giustini, 2006, 1283).

As in the past, the central problem of conducting good research is to stay abreast of developments within a field of study. Healthcare and biomedicine are areas where new developments occur in rapid succession and leaps in discovery happen. Thus, the need to stay as networked as possible and to be 'tuned in' to new developments and discoveries is essential. Web 2.0 tools and technologies offer many options for accomplishing this goal. In addition, the pathway from primary research to knowledge translation to discovery by clinicians has been greatly expedited by these tools. As Hughes et al. note in their 2009 study of the junior physician's use of Web 2.0, 'although credibility of information was the most cited concern, tools such as Wikipedia or Google are used 3 times more . . . than PubMed, the "official" best evidence tool introduced in medical school' (Hughes et al., 2009, 651).

Thus, one must choose wisely in the realm of Web 2.0 and use good information literacy skills in evaluating content, identifying its provenance and placing it in context. The new social media and networking tools can facilitate resource discovery and information retrieval to a great extent, but effectively identifying the source of such information and ensuring that high-quality, accurate information spreads through these viral networks requires vigilance. Some examples follow of Web 2.0 tools and technologies and how they can be used to support research. Where appropriate, recommendations are given as to relevance, and caveats or potential pitfalls noted.

Twitter and blogs

Blogs enable individuals to easily publish their own websites in the form of regular posts. Many researchers as well as institutions and research centres use this tool to maintain blogs with posts pertaining to ongoing research or summarizing their own new research or that of others. For example, the Mayo Clinic in the USA has a blog, http://newsblog.mayoclinic.org/, and many healthcare researchers and health librarians maintain blogs, such as Laika's MedLibLog (http://laikaspoetnik.wordpress.com/). Another excellent example of a medical research blog is Clinical Cases and Images (http://casesblog.blogspot.com/). One can take RSS feeds of blog posts from a particular blog and insert comments on posts. Thus, when aggregated into an RSS feed reader such as iGoogle or Netvibes, they provide an overview of research being conducted in a particular area.

Twitter, a so-called microblogging service, allows for the sharing of short (140 characters) messages which often include links to related background information. Users choose to follow a particular twitterer's feed. Both Twitter and traditional blogs offer an effective means of staying up to date in a particular healthcare field. As bloggers will often also have a Twitter account where they tweet links or information related to their field of study, there is often overlap between blog and Twitter posts. Tools such as Tweetdeck allow users to filter Twitter for specific keywords or hashtags (the # symbol followed by a keyword). Thus, users of these tools are able to follow developments, sometimes in real time, in a specific healthcare research area or topic.

The benefits of traditional blogs are that they are often an efficient source for summaries of research – but it can be quite time consuming to read all the posts from all the relevant blogs. Twitter, on the other hand, offers a more concise feed of information, but can easily become overwhelming if one follows too many streams. As is the case with all Web 2.0 tools, the user must strike a balance between quality of content and investment of time, and select the blogs and/or Twitter feeds that offer the best return on investment in terms of research value. And, as always, good information literacy skills are needed to ensure that the quality, accuracy and timeliness of the information provided by the selected sources are good.

Wikis and collaborative environments

Wikis and other collaborative working or research environments are an excellent example of the power of Web 2.0 tools. They offer interactive, user-generated and collaborative environments for researchers and are simple to use. Wikis (the name originates from the Hawaiian word *wiki*, meaning 'quick' or 'fast', but has also become a backronym for 'What I Know Is') are online resources that are created by many users via a process of editing and re-editing. The best known example is Wikipedia, though the paradigm has shifted into many areas, including wikis such as Medpedia (www.medpedia.com/) and the HLWiki (Health Libraries Wiki) from UC Alberta (http://hlwiki.slais.ubc.ca). As the HLWiki notes, 'while clearly useful for certain projects, wikis are not universally useful in health where standards of accuracy must attain the highest levels for human safety' (HLWiki, 2010). But the peer-reviewed nature of these resources, combined with the ease of editing content, offers great potential for enhancing the research process, especially if this is undertaken in a controlled environment. In addition to wikis, tools like Mendeley (www.mendeley.com), which are at the intersection of collaborative environments and social networking and social bookmarking, offer similar potential with regard to supporting research.

While the quality of the information in wikis and other collaborative online resources is most often very high, again, one must always fact-check the sources and remain vigilant with respect to the provenance of information in these resources. This is especially pertinent given that 'Wikipedia ranked among the first ten results in 71–85% of search engines and keywords tested [surpassing] MedlinePlus and NHS Direct Online ... and ranked higher with quality articles' in a study by Hughes et al. (2009). The ease with which these resources can be used to share and add knowledge to the research environment means that they are likely to be a relevant source for research for the foreseeable future.

Social networking

On the face of it, an idea like online social networking seems an obvious choice for enhancing the research process. Researchers have always tried to network by attending conferences, peer-reviewing papers, joining organizations and societies and other networking activities. Thus, the notion of using Facebook or more research-oriented social networking tools like 2Collab (www.2collab.com/), ResearchGate (www.researchgate.net/) or Nature Network (http://network.nature.com/) should not be a novel one. Social networking tools offer basic features such as creating profiles and sharing links and information, and often provide communication tools such as chat and favouring or 'liking' posts. No other Web 2.0 tool marshals what appear to be somewhat trite activities in useful and effective ways for networking with peers and colleagues.

Facebook, currently the largest social networking site on the web, was originally intended as a way for friends and family to stay connected. However, it has evolved into a platform whereby any group of individuals interested in a particular topic, say a research area in healthcare, can connect, share and interact via wall posts, sharing links and documents, and organizing events. The use of Facebook for professional networking and its overlap with an individual's personal life has flagged some risks with regard to posting or sharing unprofessional content. As Chretien et al. note, 'the social contract between medicine and society expects physicians to embody altruism, integrity, and trustworthiness [and] furthermore, ethical and legal obligations to maintain patient confidentiality have unique repercussions' in healthcare (Chretien et al., 2009, 1309). So, care must be taken to ensure that privacy settings and other measures are in place to secure a researcher's online identity and that they are seen as acting appropriately in these spheres.

As mentioned above, other social networking tools offer a more targeted approach for researchers and scientists. Sites like 2Collab enable researchers 'to share, connect and discuss relevant research with your peers'. Similarly, ResearchGate, which claims to have over 500,000 scientific members, allows for such features as building your own scientific network, collaborating on projects and finding conferences and even jobs. The most recently established social network comes from *Nature* magazine and is called Nature Network. It offers researchers space to maintain their own blogs, connect with other researchers and participate in forums and join groups, among other features. As these types of services have a research focus, the issues of posting inappropriate content and other ethical concerns associated with Facebook or more generic social networking sites are less worrisome. Taken together, social networking and social bookmarking offer effective, time-saving tools for conducting research.

Social bookmarking

Social bookmarking tools were some of the first widely adopted Web 2.0 tools, and for obvious reasons. They offer an easy way to tag, manage and share what sites or pages individuals visit on the web. The social nature of these bookmarking services enables researchers to see what others are reading and to share references. In addition, there is a very practical reason why social bookmarking tools have grown in popularity on the web: they offer an easy way to store all of your bookmarks on a web-based platform that can be accessed from any computer. Also, widgets and plug-ins for popular browsers such as Firefox make it effortless to add bookmarks to an account on these services.

Delicious (www.delicious.com/) was one of the first widely used social bookmarking sites. Account creation is simple and the service offers a flexible tagging system and options for integration with other Web 2.0 tools, such as Facebook, and plug-ins for most browsers. CiteULike (www.citeulike.org/) and Connotea (www.connotea.org/) offer a more research-centred approach to the social bookmarking paradigm. Connotea labels itself as 'free online reference management for all researchers, clinicians and scientists', while CiteULike describes itself as a 'free service for managing and discovering scholarly references'. Both offer researchers the opportunity to peer inside others' bookmarks and reading lists and they provide user-friendly platforms for organizing references and exporting citations in various formats such as BibTeX and EndNote for use in scholarly papers. Social bookmarking tools, especially those with a scholarly or research focus, are an efficient way for busy researchers to organize their references.

RSS and 'push' technologies

A discussion of RSS and 'push' technologies is a logical way to wrap up a discussion of Web 2.0 and how it supports research, as these technologies really bring it all together for users. RSS, usually spelled out as Really Simple Syndication, is an XML standard that provides an easy way to subscribe to a feed of content from a website or online service. The content can be news stories, blog posts, new journal articles, audio content (usually podcasts), video content or any other kind of published data on the web. RSS is often called a 'push' technology – in contrast to the Web 1.0 idea of having to 'pull' content from websites – because previously defined content is 'pushed' to the user via RSS feeds that are aggregated into a variety of platforms and services (such as iGoogle, see below) that the user can access. The obvious implication for a researcher is that relevant content is received automatically rather than having to be retrieved directly from websites.

A related phenomenon that is often powered by RSS takes the form of services that allow users to create their own home pages or 'dashboards' for the web content they are interested in. For example, iGoogle (www.google.com/ig) allows users with Google accounts to organize all of their RSS feeds into a single home page. Netvibes (www.netvibes.com) takes this paradigm a step further and offers users the ability to create a range of dashboards for organizing content from a variety of sources (RSS feeds, Twitterfeeds, social networking friendfeeds, etc.). More specifically for health and medicine researchers, services like Webicina's PeRSSonalized Medicine (www.webicina.com/perssonalized/) offer 'a free, easy-to-use aggregator of quality medical information that lets users select their favorite resources and read the latest news and articles about a medical specialty or a medical condition in a personalized space' (Webicina, 2010). Taking the paradigm even further, MedWorm (www.medworm.com/) serves as a kind of meta-RSS feed generator, and is described on the site as the medical router of the internet where 'over 6000 authoritative RSS feeds go in / hundreds of new RSS feeds by category come out'. Regardless of the service used, the paradigm of having content 'pushed' at oneself rather than having to go laboriously searching for it holds great appeal for busy researchers.

Summary

Web 2.0 tools and technologies offer a range of new and innovative options and paradigms for supporting research in healthcare and biomedicine, each with its own benefits and potential pitfalls. Blogs and Twitter offer a user-friendly way to follow others' research while enabling easy self-publishing of one's own content. Wikis and collaborative working environments offer a more engaging medium for contributing to the research process via simple web-based editing and publishing. Social networking and social bookmarking bring together researchers with similar interests into online networks that enable sharing, collaboration and learning from each other's work. Finally, RSS and 'push' technologies and their related aggregation tools offer a way to bring it all together and to customize and streamline the process of consuming content online. But, just as with any information retrieval tool or resource, appropriate information literacy skills need to be used to determine factors such as authority, provenance and accuracy, especially with regard to health and biomedical information. Web 2.0 both enables good, high-quality information to spread fast and allows for bad information to go viral. However, with diligence and a keen attention to these issues, navigating this new social web landscape can greatly enhance the research process.

References and further reading

Chretien, K. et al. (2009) Online Posting of Unprofessional Content by Medical Students, *JAMA*, **302** (12), 1309–15.

Ginn, S. (2010) Evidence Based Mental Health and Web 2.0, *Evidence-Based Mental Health*, **13** (3), 69–72.

Giustini, D. (2006) How Web 2.0 is Changing Medicine: is a medical wikipedia the next step? *BMJ*, **333**, 1283–4.

HLWiki (2010) *Using Web 2.0 Tools in Health Research*, UBC, http://hlwiki.slais.ubc.ca/index.php/Using_web_2.0_tools_in_health_research_at_UBC.

Hughes, B., Joshi, I., Lemonde, H. and Wareham, J. (2009) Junior Physician's Use of Web 2.0 for Information Seeking and Medical Education: a qualitative study, *International Journal of Medical Informatics*, **78**, 645–55.

Sharp, J. (2008) Web 2.0 in Clinical Research, *Slideshare*, www.slideshare.net/JohnSharp/web-20-in-clinical-research.

Webicina (2010) *PeRSSonalized Medicine*, www.webicina.com/perssonalized/.

Wright, A. (2008) Creating and Sharing Clinical Decision Support Content with Web 2.0: issues and examples, *Journal of Biomedical Informatics*, **42**, 334–46.

CHAPTER 6

Crowdsourcing: the identification of content suitable for the developing world

Jon Brassey

Introduction: what is crowdsourcing?

According to Wikipedia (http://en.wikipedia.org/wiki/Crowdsourcing):

> Crowdsourcing is a neologistic compound of 'crowd' and 'outsourcing' for the act of outsourcing tasks, traditionally performed by an employee or contractor to a large group of people or community (a crowd), through an open call.

In other words, you take a long-winded or complex task (that a computer typically cannot do well), break it down into smaller packets of work and get a group of people (the crowd) to each take a packet and work through it.

The most prominent recent example of crowdsourcing was the search for the American adventurer Steve Fossett. He went missing whilst flying over the Nevada desert on 3 September 2007. He hadn't filed a flight plan, so his aeroplane could have been anywhere within a 4- to 5-hour flying radius of the private airstrip known as Flying-M Ranch. On 8 September the first of a series of new high-resolution imagery was made available via the Amazon Mechanical Turk beta website so that users could flag potential areas of interest to be searched (http://en.wikipedia.org/wiki/Steve_Fossett#Disappearance_and_search). The area was broken down into 300,000 squares, each measuring 278 feet square and covering the area where it was believed Fossett might have crashed. The principle in use was that users should look at individual squares for any signs of plane wreckage. By 11 September, up to 50,000 people had joined the effort and it was understood that each square had been viewed at least once. Unfortunately, there was no happy ending and on 29 October the site was closed, without any measurable success.

Other examples of crowdsourcing include: Facebook, using this approach to help create different language versions of the site; *The Guardian* newspaper's investigation into the MPs' expenses affair in the UK (users sifted through 700,000 expenses claim forms); and, arguably, Wikipedia itself.

There have been some examples of using crowdsourcing in the medical world, but few have a high profile. Perhaps the most prominent is Medpedia (www.medpedia.

com/), which is a medical version of Wikipedia. Amongst other prominent initiatives that include an element of crowdsourcing are PatientsLikeMe (www.patientslikeme.com/) and the People's Open Access Education Initiative (http://peoples-uni.org/).

The TRIP Database and the problem of the developing world

The TRIP Database was established in 1997 as a simple, crudely searchable repository of secondary reviews of the evidence (e.g. systematic reviews, clinical guidelines). After it received some early attention in *Bandolier* (Anonymous, 1998) usage and functionality of the database increased significantly. From its initial focus we (those of us involved in running the TRIP Database) became increasingly aware that secondary reviews of the primary research evidence only answered a relatively small number of clinical questions (in our experience between 20–25%). Those of us involved in compiling and maintaining the TRIP Database made the choice that the primary focus was to help clinicians find answers to their questions using the best available evidence. In other words, if there were no secondary reviews, then primary research and e-textbooks should be included. Further developments were stimulated by both spontaneous (Montori and Ebbert, 2002) and commissioned reviews (Meats et al. 2007). The database is currently searched approximately one million times per month and has a worldwide audience. While the majority of the searches come from 'western' nations, approximately 12% of users reside in the developing world.

Irrespective of the technical merits of the TRIP Database, searching is frequently problematic. Users are frequently unskilled in their searching methods, with the most popular searches being single-term searches on topics such as hypertension, asthma and diabetes. These return large numbers of results and the user then has to spend a significant amount of time looking through the results list to find the answer to their question. Users from the developing world find that many of the interventions are not available, due to resource constraints. So, not only do they have to search through a wide set of results, but in addition, many of the interventions highlighted are not suitable for their setting (Chinnock, Siegfried and Clarke, 2005; World Health Organisation, 2005).

The problems of access to research evidence have been highlighted by a number of different organizations and much of the effort of highlighting the problems of access to the research evidence by those in the developing world has been focused by the umbrella campaign Health Information For All 2015 (HIFA2015, www.hifa2015.org). In their 2004 article in *The Lancet*, Fiona Godlee et al. reported:

> Universal access to information for health professionals is a prerequisite for meeting the Millennium Development Goals and achieving Health for All. However, despite the promises of the information revolution, and some successful initiatives, there is little if any evidence that the majority of health professionals in the developing world are any better informed than they were 10 years ago. Lack of access to information remains a major barrier to knowledge-based health care in developing countries.

To promote access to pertinent health information, the problem was how to identify a corpus of content, contained within the TRIP index. This was beyond the ability of computers to do, in other words a program could not be written to identify content suitable for the developing world. And so, the idea of crowdsourcing was explored. We spoke with a number of people from a variety of settings, including the World Health Organisation (WHO) and HINARI (the Health InterNetwork Access to Research Initiative, set up by WHO and major publishers to enable developing countries to access collections of biomedical and health literature, www.who.int/hinari/en/), HIFA2015 and the American National Library of Medicine. This was so as to both better understand the issues relating to access to information and also determine whether our suggested methodology might be suitable.

The initial concept of using crowdsourcing received considerable support, which helped in further refinement of the idea. In addition, a grant was made available from BUPA's charitable giving initiative, BUPA Giving. (BUPA is a UK-based private healthcare organization which has recently diversified into a global brand and is now an internationally established provider of health insurance and care.)

For the system to work it needed to be simple and easy to use. A clickable link was added under each result, stating 'Developing World?' If a user believed an article was suitable for the developing world they simply clicked on the link and that article would receive a 'vote'. An article would only be added to the corpus of 'developing world' articles if it received a minimum of two clicks from different people; this was to avoid an article being added to the corpus by someone accidentally clicking twice on a link.

At the same time as the 'Developing World?' link was implemented under each result on the TRIP Database, a tick box was introduced within the search filter section of the results page, labelled 'Suitable for the Developing World'. When a user searches, they can tick this box and only those results deemed suitable for the developing world (by having already received two clicks) will be shown.

Progress to date

At the time of writing, the service has been running for a little over two months and a total of 135 articles have received two clicks and are thus part of the corpus of articles deemed suitable for the developing world. In addition, over 450 articles have received one click. A search for *hypertension* on the TRIP Database finds over 33,000 articles; restricting that search to 'developing world' shows ten results. The top three results for the main search are:

- Interventions used to improve control of blood pressure in patients with hypertension (Cochrane Database of Systematic Reviews)
- Primary prevention of CVD: treating hypertension (*Clinical Evidence*)
- Roselle for hypertension in adults (Cochrane Database of Systematic Reviews).

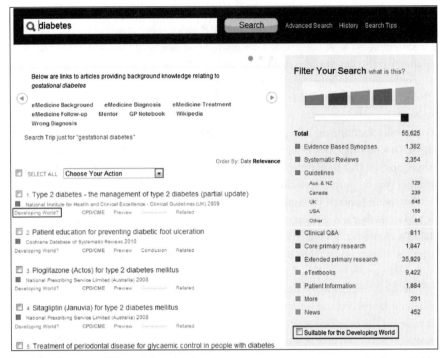

Figure 6.1 *A screenshot of the TRIP Database results page with the Developing World functionality highlighted*

Compare that to when the 'developing world' filter is applied:

- Placental malarial infection as a risk factor for hypertensive disorders during pregnancy in Africa: a case-control study in an urban area of Senegal, West Africa (*American Journal of Epidemiology*)
- Cost-effectiveness analysis of hypertension guidelines in South Africa: absolute risk versus blood pressure level (NHS Economic Evaluation Database)
- Hypertension in sub-Saharan Africa: a systematic review (*Hypertension*).

In the case of a search for *diabetes* the results are over 55,500, versus 11 relevant to the developing world (Figure 6.1). Again, comparing the two search modes shows that the top three results for the main search are:

- Type 2 diabetes – the management of type 2 diabetes (National Institute for Health and Clinical Excellence)
- Patient education for preventing diabetic foot ulceration (Cochrane Database of Systematic Reviews)
- Pioglitazone (Actos) for type 2 diabetes mellitus (National Prescribing Service Limited).

While the results when the 'developing world' filter is applied are:

- Hypoglycaemic activity of four plant extracts traditionally used in South Africa for diabetes (*Journal of Ethnopharmacology*)
- An effective system of nurse-led diabetes care in rural Africa (*Diabetic Medicine*)
- Burden of diabetic illness in an urban hospital in Nigeria (*Tropical Doctor*).

The low number of developing world results highlights that the service is still very new and has a long way to go. It is highly likely that there are a significant number of articles within the TRIP Database that have yet to be identified using crowdsourcing, thus limiting the usefulness of the service at the present time. Over time, more articles will become highlighted, making the service more useful.

On a positive note, all the articles currently highlighted are appropriate, suggesting that the technique has real potential.

Lessons learned

Perhaps the biggest difficulty faced when developing the idea of applying crowdsourcing was the branding, and this was most apparent with the naming. A system needed to be developed that would be immediately recognizable and usable.

To give it greater prominence, it was felt that the prompt (the 'Developing World?' link) had to be shown under each search result, and therefore it needed to be short and direct. Initially, the designers turned to the idea of a globe icon on which Africa and other resource-poor regions were highlighted. However, when this was repeated under each result it dominated the results page and drew attention away from the actual results. It was therefore decided to use a textual link (matching other existing textual links, e.g. for related articles). With regard to the wording, there was conflicting advice. While the term 'Developing World' was eventually used, it became clear that this was controversial. Some of the organizations we spoke to indicated that a more appropriate term would have been 'suitable for resource-poor settings', their argument being that our initiative highlighted low-cost interventions and this excluded some developing-world situations and included some developed-world situations. However, we felt that this was long-winded (space is at a premium on our results pages) and we also felt it was confusing for most users of the TRIP Database.

Also, as most of the users of the TRIP Database come from the 'developed' world it was felt that the term 'developing world' was more meaningful and instantly recognizable. The fact that the WHO uses the term provided significant support for the decision. However, it was decided to keep an open mind and possibly to replace the term 'developing world' with another if the consensus was that it needed to be replaced.

Also, promotion of the service could have been (and could still be) better. During the creation of the initiative we spoke with a large number of people and found almost universal encouragement and goodwill. We could have better enrolled these people as promoters of the service to their respective audiences. I also think, given the large number of users of the TRIP Database, that we could do better at signposting the initiative. We do mention it in a number of places on the site (e.g. under each result, on the home page and at the top of the results page), but it could be stronger or clearer. However, that raises another issue that affects most websites – the limited screen 'real estate'. With a limited screen size and possibly many features to highlight, there is a tension between those features that gain most prominence and those that have a lesser role.

Conclusions

Irrespective of the potential shortcomings raised above, I feel that crowdsourcing is still valid and has shown itself to be useful and worthwhile. In starting to work in this area we have been guided by a large number of enthusiastic and gifted individuals who have opened up possibilities for taking this work forward. These relationships have opened up a number of possible additional uses for the output, including in an African continuing professional development initiative using mobile phones as part of a wider content delivery scheme. We are also in the early stages of an additional crowdsourcing initiative allowing clinicians to record and share their learning with each other. While not specific to resource-poor settings the new initiative lends itself to mobile technology and so has many possible applications. The topic area – highlighting evidence suitable for the developing world – is so important that efforts must be made to meet a clear need. Any solution is likely to be multi-factorial and our crowdsourcing approach could have a significant role to play.

References

Anonymous (1998) Searching for Evidence – TRIP Database, *Bandolier*, **49**, http://www.medicine.ox.ac.uk/bandolier/band49/b49ads.html#Heading3.

Chinnock, P., Siegfried, N. and Clarke, M. (2005) Is Evidence-Based Medicine Relevant to the Developing World? *Evidence-based Complementary and Alternative Medicine*, **2** (3), 321–4.

Godlee, F., Pakenham-Walsh, N., Ncayiyana, D., Cohen, B. and Packer, A. (2004) Can We Achieve Health Information for All by 2015? *Lancet*, **364** (9430), 295–300.

Meats, E., Brassey, J., Heneghan, C. and Glasziou, P. (2007) Using the Turning Research Into Practice (TRIP) Database: how do clinicians really search? *Journal of the Medical Library Association*, **95** (2), 156–63.

Montori, V. M. and Ebbert, J. O. (2002) TRIP database, *ACP Journal Club*, **137** (1), A15.

World Health Organisation (2005) *Knowledge Management Strategy*, World Health Organisation, www.who.int/kms/about/strategy/en/.

CHAPTER 7

Supporting patient needs: an overview of the potential role of Web 2.0 in patient and consumer information

Paula Younger

Introduction

The ultimate aims of healthcare information are to provide information, whether mediated or directly, and to allow patients or health consumers to maintain a good level of health, manage an existing condition or prevent conditions worsening.

Under the NHS Constitution, information provision is now a legal right for patients in the UK. Patients have the right to 'be given information about [the] proposed treatment in advance, including any significant risks and any alternative treatments which may be available, and the risks involved in doing nothing'. In addition, patients have the right 'to be involved in discussions and decisions about your healthcare, and to be given information to enable...this' (Department of Health, 2010).

Web 2.0 would seem to represent a perfect platform for providing patient or consumer information and support for public health in general, offering new, innovative, cost-effective, responsive and timely ways in which to provide that information.

What sources do patients use for information?

In the UK, patients attending their GP surgery (family practitioner) or being discharged from hospital will often be given an information leaflet about their condition which may or may not include details of websites. There are some excellent websites, such as www.patient.co.uk. Many charities also provide a wide range of well researched information, often available for free download from their websites. When medicines are purchased, whether on prescription or over the counter, information leaflets are provided in the packaging.

Some dissatisfaction has been expressed by patients regarding the information they receive from medical and healthcare professionals, nonetheless (Kinnersley et al., 2008). Further, studies suggest that although many patients use health websites that have been put together by government-backed organizations, such as NHS Direct and the BBC, these sites do not necessarily meet their needs (Huntington et al., 2007). In future, however, the way in which patients and health consumers receive their health information may well be through a computer-mediated avatar (Van den Brekel, 2007).

What is of consequence to us as potential mediators of information, then, is the reason why patients would turn to the Web 2.0 realm for health information. Change appears to be taking place in many areas: on the one hand, there is distrust of authority and experts; on the other, an information explosion has been made possible by modern information and communication technologies (Lor and General, 2008). Healthcare professionals regularly express concern about the quality and veracity of health information on the internet in general, but do not necessarily ask themselves why patients may not find the information provided by hospital or physician sources adequate for their needs.

Patient information needs

Patient information needs may vary, depending on whether their condition is acute or chronic, and on the nature of their condition or situation. In some studies, only 20% of patients overall had sought health information online; those in poor health, were 10 to 13 times more likely to have participated in online support forums (Huntington et al., 2004). The need for any information provision to be patient-centred remains clear (Pulman, 2010), as does the low level of confidence in many web-based sites (Berman, 2010). Recent changes in UK legislation have strengthened the right of patients to receive information that will enable them to make an informed decision about their care (Smith and Duman, 2009).

Blogs and wikis

There are many blogs available for patients, such as expert patient blogs on the topics of cancer or diabetes. Where they are well researched and well policed they can offer an excellent opportunity for patients to interact and gain information (Nordfeldt et al., 2010). In many ways, online blogs simply represent a virtual version of the long-established support group, as is apparent from the subject areas covered, such as pain management and smoking cessation (Graham et al., 2009; Hasman and Chiarella, 2008). The potentially healing aspect of writing about a condition has also been identified (Kim, 2009).

The personalized patient

Another way in which Web 2.0 can be used to support patients is via personalized start pages on the internet. With Web 2.0 applications such as mashups, it is possible to set up a home page with links that are directly relevant to the user. For a condition such as diabetes, for example, a mashup could incorporate RSS feeds from journals or charities, information about the latest research, advice on nutrition and a BMI calculator. This move towards a more personalized and responsive healthcare information system for patients has been highlighted as desirable by many authors (Abidi and Goh, 2001), particularly for the way in which it hands over knowledge about healthcare to the patient (Gardiner, 2008). Ultimately, it will be possible for patients to have home-based personalized healthcare.

Have you had your Tweet today? The use of social media in patient information

With over half the world's population using mobile phones (Beaumont, 2009), text messaging is potentially an extremely cost-effective method of reaching a high proportion of patients. Twitter represents the next development. Whether social media should be used to communicate with patients raises some ethical questions, however, particularly relating to confidentiality and security of patient data.

Other potential uses for social media in patient information include notifying patients about events, offering tutorials and carrying out surveys (Boyd and Ellison, 2007). Many health organizations, ranging from the British Heart Foundation to Norfolk and Norwich University Hospitals NHS Foundation Trust, now have Facebook pages and use their pages for just those kinds of notification.

Patient records and information

One of the major concerns about using Web 2.0 to deliver information to patients relates to the security and confidentiality of patient records (Moszynski, 2008). Even if information is anecdotal, as healthcare information professionals, we must pay attention to the requirements of data protection and try to ensure that our users are equally aware of the risks. One solution might be to implement secure patient portals, as described by Nehring (c.2011).

The doctor–patient relationship through Web 2.0

Web 2.0 is changing the nature of the way in which doctors and patients interact. Patients are now very likely to research their own condition on the internet, whether via forums, wikis, blogs, or other resources. Little research, however, has been done into levels of health literacy amongst patients (Smith and Duman, 2009) and, as some clinicians and healthcare providers fear, a little knowledge can be a dangerous thing (Hurley and Smith, 2007).

The two-way nature of Web 2.0 could also be utilized to great effect by healthcare professionals to establish the concerns of patients suffering from particular conditions or to correct erroneous information. Concerns are regularly expressed about the quality of the information, but there appears to be relatively little understanding of the fact that, for the majority of patients, much information provided by the healthcare establishment is too technical and lacks the personal touch.

Reaching hard-to-reach patients

One of the most attractive aspects of many Web 2.0 applications is their potential to reach those who may not necessarily approach traditional healthcare providers. These groups include the disabled, the housebound, those in rural areas, the socially disadvantaged, adolescents and men.

Public Health

The area of public health is also one where Web 2.0 can potentially be extremely useful in what Eysenbach describes as 'infodemiology' (2008). So far, Twitter has been used in times of disaster to both inform the rest of the world about events and reassure loved ones of the safety of survivors.

Web 2.0 applications have also been used to track epidemics, and could potentially be used to target healthcare resources and inform the public in times of national disaster. The CDC (Centers for Disease Control and Prevention), for example, issued alerts on Twitter about health issues related to the Gulf of Mexico oil spill in 2010.

The role of libraries and healthcare information professionals

Historically, librarians appear to have had relatively little input into the provision of patient information, although this may be on the verge of changing. There have, however, been some very encouraging recent examples of joint projects between public libraries and more specialized healthcare libraries (Brettle, 2008).

As information professionals, we can envisage contributing to patient information in many ways. These include assisting with health literacy programmes; working in partnership with other organizations; and supporting our healthcare and medical professionals to make the information available in an authoritative way.

References and further reading

Abidi, S. S. R. and Goh, A. (2001) A Personalised Healthcare Information Delivery System: pushing customised healthcare information over the WWW. In Hasman, A., Blobel, B., Dudeck, J., Engelbrecht, R., Gell, G. and Prokosch, H. (eds), *Medical Infobahn in Europe (MIE'2000)*, IOS Press, http://web.cs.dal.ca/~sraza/papers/MIE00_PHI.pdf.

Beaumont, C. (2009) Half of World's Population Owns a Mobile Phone, UN Study Reveals, *Daily Telegraph*, (3 March), www.telegraph.co.uk/technology/news/4933263/Half-of-worlds-population-owns-a-mobile-phone-UN-study-reveals.html.

Berman, M. R. (2010) The Sorry State of US Government Consumer Health Information, *medpage today*, (24 September), www.medpagetoday.com/Blogs/22332.

Boyd, D. and Ellison, N. (2007) Social Network Sites: definition, history, and

scholarship, *Journal of Computer-Mediated Communication*, **13** (1),
http://jcmc.indiana.edu/vol13/issue1/boyd.ellison.html.

Brawn, T. S. (2005) Consumer Health Libraries: what do patrons really want? *Journal of the Medical Library Association*, **93** (4), 495–9.

Brettle, A. and Ormandy, P. (2008) *Do NHS Libraries have a Role in Providing Patient Information?*, University of Salford, http://usir.salford.ac.uk/3151/1/Brettle_A_NHS_Libraries_Final_Report_Oct_2008_FINAL.pdf.

Brettle, A., Hulme, C. T. and Ormandy, P. (2005) *Effective Methods of Providing Information for Patient Care (EMPIRIC Project): Report Three – Data Collection and Analysis*, University of Salford, Health Care Practice R&D Unit, http://www.nursing.salford.ac.uk/research_dev/EMPIRIC%20Literature%20Review.pdf.

Department of Health (2010) *The NHS Constitution*, Department of Health, www.nhs.uk/choiceintheNHS/Rightsandpledges/NHSConstitution/Documents/nhs-constitution-interactive-version-march-2010.pdf.

Eysenbach, G. (2008) *Infodemiology and Infoveillance*, www.slideshare.net/eysen/infodemiology-infoveillance-twitter-and-googlebased-surveillance-the-infovigil-system.

Fulda, P. O. and Kwasik, H. (2004) Consumer Health Information Provided by Library and Other Hospital Websites in the South Central Region, *Journal of the Medical Library Association*, **92** (3), 372–7.

Gardiner, R. (2008) The Transition from 'Informed Patient' Care to 'Patient Informed' Care, *Studies in Health Technology and Informatics*, **137**, 241.

Graham, C., Rouncefield, M. and Satchell, C. (2009) Blogging as 'Therapy'? Exploring personal technologies for smoking cessation, *Health Informatics Journal*, **15** (4), 267–81.

Hammond, P.A. (2005) Consumer Health Librarian, *Reference Services Review*, **33** (1), 38–43.

Hasman, L. and Chiarella, D. (2008) Developing a Pain Management Resource Wiki for Cancer Patients and Their Caregivers, *Journal of Consumer Health on the Internet*, **12** (4), 317–26.

Huntington, P., Nicholas, D., Homewood, J., Polydoratou, P., Gunter, B., Russell, C. and Withey, R. (2004) The General Public's Use of (and attitudes towards) Interactive, Personal Digital Health Information and Advisory Services, *Journal of Documentation*, **60** (3), 245–65.

Huntington, P., Nicholas, D., Jamali, H. R. and Russell, C. (2007) Health Information for the Consumer: NHS vs the BBC, *Aslib Proceedings*, **59** (1), 46–67.

Hurley, M. and Smith, C. (2007) Patients' Blogs – Do Doctors Have Anything to Fear?, *BMJ*, **335** (7621), 645–6.

Kim, S. (2009) Content Analysis of Cancer Blog Posts, *Journal of the Medical Library Association*, **97** (4), 260–6.

Kinnersley, P., Edwards, A. G. K., Hood, K., Cadbury, N., Ryan, R., Prout, H., Owen, D., MacBeth, F., Butow, P. and Butler, C. (2008) Interventions before

Consultations for Helping Patients Address Their Information Needs, *BMJ*, **337**, a485.

Laurent, M. R. and Vickers, T. J. (2009) Seeking Health Information Online: does Wikipedia matter? *Journal of the American Medical Informatics Association*, **16** (4), 471–9.

Leithner, A., Maurer-Ertl, W., Glehr, M., Friesenbichler, J., Leithner, K. and Windhager, R. (2010) Wikipedia and Osteosarcoma: a trustworthy patients' information? *Journal of the American Medical Informatics Association*, **17** (4), 373–4.

Lor, P. and General, S. (2008) International Librarianship 2.0: some international dimensions of Web 2.0 and Library 2.0. *VALA 2008 Conference*, www.valaconf.org.au/vala2008/papers2008/154_Lor_Keynote_Final.pdf.

Moszynski, P. (2008) Study Highlights Risk of Breaking Patient Confidentiality in Blogs, *BMJ*, **337** (7764), 254–5.

Nehring, G. (c.2011) Patient Portals: a jumpstart on meeting meaningful use requirements, *HIMSS News*, www.himss.org/ASP/ ContentRedirector.asp?ContentId=74627&type=HIMSSNewsItem.

Nordfeldt, S., Hanberger, L. and Berterö, C. (2010) Patient and Parent Views on a Web 2.0 Diabetes Portal – the Management Tool, the Generator, and the Gatekeeper: qualitative study, *Journal of Medical Internet Research*, **12** (2), e17, http://www.ncbi.nlm.nih.gov/pmc/articles/PMC2956228/?tool=pubmed.

Pulman, A. (2010) A Patient Centred Framework for Improving LTC Quality of Life Through Web 2.0 Technology, *Health Informatics Journal*, **16** (1), 15–23.

Ruffin, A. B., Cogdill, K., Kutty, L. and Hudson-Ochillo, M. (2005) Access to Electronic Health Information for the Public: analysis of fifty three funded projects, *Library Trends*, **53** (3), 434–51.

Smith, S. and Duman, M. (2009) The State of Consumer Health Information: an overview, *Health Information and Libraries Journal*, **26** (4), 260–78.

Van den Brekel, A. (2007) *Get Your Consumer Health Information from an Avatar! Health and medical related activities in a virtual environment*, www.slideshare.net/digicmb/ getting-your-consumer-health-information-from-an-avatar.

CHAPTER 8

Some ethical and legal considerations in the use of Web 2.0

Peter Morgan

Introduction

Like all professionals, librarians and other information specialists are subject both to ethical standards that guide their professional conduct, and to legal regulation. It would be entirely wrong to suppose that the growth of the internet is solely responsible for determining the nature of the obligations and constraints to which professional behaviour is nowadays expected to conform. Many of these principles have been with us for far longer, establishing lasting social values and responsibilities that are fundamentally just as relevant now as they ever were. Issues such as copyright, defamation and negligence – and the need to be aware of them – were part of the fabric of professional life long before the internet arrived.

The new society of the internet

It is also true, however, that the internet's development has made a significant difference in at least two respects. First, it has accelerated the pace of technology-driven change, and in so doing has forced us to reconsider whether the existing ethical and legal framework is still adequate. When Charlie Chaplin (commenting on moral issues created by the emergence of atomic weapons) wrote 'Man is an animal with primary instincts of survival. Consequently, his ingenuity has developed first and his soul afterwards. Thus the progress of science is far ahead of man's ethical behaviour' (Chaplin, 1964, 507), he was drawing attention to the same relentless process of technological change and human response. Present-day examples can be seen in the public debates surrounding *in vitro* fertilization, genetic modification and stem-cell research. So it is inevitable that the all-pervasive growth of the internet's influence should be followed by a reassessment and redefinition of the standards we need to adopt in order to exploit it responsibly, and we need to be aware of how the results affect our professional activities.

This leads to the second difference, and one that perhaps uniquely defines the internet's character. Kevan and McGrath (2001) describe it thus: 'The relationship between law and the internet is based upon a simple conflict: laws exist to regulate society; [but] the internet has created a new society founded upon the principle that it should be wholly unregulated.' The consequences of that 'simple conflict' are in fact anything but simple, and contain further complexities that are relevant to us. First, the international nature of internet communications and the 'internet society' means that the legal framework governing them is subject not only to the laws of each individual country in which internet-based activity takes place, but also to the growing number of transnational agreements such as those formulated by the European Community – and the different jurisdictions cannot always be reconciled. At the opposite end of the spectrum from issues of international governance are those relating to the role of the individual. The participative nature of the internet encourages us to use it in both professional and social life. We therefore become proficient in using its various services and tools for a wide range of purposes; but in so doing, we may deliberately or unintentionally blur the distinction between what we do in a professional capacity and what we do on a personal basis. If we fail to understand or respect the distinction, and if we then find ourselves defending a complaint from an aggrieved third party, such as may happen following a contentious e-mail message, blog post, or tweet that we believed was being published in a personal capacity, we may nonetheless be involving both ourselves and our employer in questions of liability. And while this chapter is primarily a discussion of what might happen in a professional capacity, it cannot completely exclude the personal element.

The Web 2.0 snare

The reader will already have realized that what has been stated above is not exclusively applicable to Web 2.0, but is relevant to a far broader and longer-established set of occupational circumstances. Even so, it is possible to assert that Web 2.0 has prompted a renewed interest in many of these issues. There are several reasons for this. First, the set of tools that are generally regarded as the embodiment of Web 2.0 have appeared within a relatively short time frame, over a decade or so, and the legislative response is struggling to keep pace. This is hardly surprising if we recall the protracted saga of successive attempts at refining copyright legislation throughout the latter part of the 20th century, as the law attempted to adjust to what, with hindsight, seem like relatively modest advances in reprographic photocopier technology. Second, it is commonly observed that we live in an increasingly litigious society, one in which the consequences of a momentary lapse may result in an expensive and time-consuming process of complaint, contest and, possibly, conviction or compensation. The large number of information professionals who are routinely exploiting Web 2.0 in the course of their work may very well increase the statistical likelihood that some will transgress and be pursued in the courts; but the many different forms of exploitation that Web 2.0 can facilitate may enmesh the legal process in a succession of uncertainties regarding interpretations of the law: What exactly does 'publication' mean? In precisely which country does an internet-based offence occur? Who owns the content of a mashup? In a Web 2.0 environment the targets are frequently ill-defined or constantly moving.

Third, the culture of sharing that is the essence of Web 2.0 has focused renewed attention on protection of intellectual property and on digital rights management. Commercial organizations have become increasingly vocal in expressing their concerns, as they see their business models and profits, and therefore their incentives to be innovative, threatened by uncontrolled distribution of their commodities. Governments and inter-governmental organizations in turn are responding by adopting a less permissive attitude, drafting legislation that favours the commercial interest, and in consequence may impose deliberate or unintended restrictions on the ways in which information – the commodity in which we deal as information professionals – can be managed. And lastly, for many people Web 2.0 is not merely a set of useful applications: it represents an ideology, an opportunity to work and communicate in a more interactive, informal, transparent and immediate fashion than has ever been possible hitherto. In identifying with this aspiration and applying the 'do-it-yourself' spirit that accompanies much Web 2.0 activity, the enthusiast may be reluctant to adopt a cautious approach, preferring instead to take risks in pursuit of a goal that seems readily achievable – to act first and seek forgiveness as and when necessary.

Minimizing risks

To minimize the risks that exist in the world of Web 2.0, the healthcare information professional needs to be aware of the most likely pitfalls, and to have a clear understanding of what constitutes good practice. Thus it will be sensible to start by compiling a checklist of the legal issues that might arise, and then to consider how significant each is and what measures can be taken to eliminate the risk, or at the very least to minimize it to the point where the likely risk is deemed acceptable.

What are the likely problem areas? A basic list of legal issues would include data protection and privacy, defamation, copyright and intellectual property, negligence and breach of duty of care, accessibility, the respective liabilities of the host organization and any third-party organizations that might be engaged, and potential conflicts between national and international law. And in assessing the potential consequences of failure to anticipate and manage these risks adequately, the adverse outcomes will not be confined to possible punishment through the courts. There may also be significant risks to the organization, such as reputational damage, operational disruption through loss of data, costly rectification processes and lowering of staff morale. Kelly (2010) has provided a useful overview of how the organization might plan to identify and assess the risks, especially when a third-party service is under consideration.

The risks may apply to one, several, or all Web 2.0 applications, but a few examples will help to illustrate the problems that might arise. Blogging and Twitter have both attracted much attention, both from the media and in legal circles, because of the ease with which an innocent and well intentioned activity may become contentious and result in accusations of defamation. From the outset of blogging, its history has involved many enthusiastic adopters who were motivated by the opportunities for free expression (and in the USA, at least, could cite the First Amendment in their defence). Controversial opinions have been published as a matter of routine, and inevitably have sometimes resulted in accusations of defamation when they have overstepped the bounds of what is regarded as acceptable. The speed with which a blogged opinion is transmitted, and the fact that it may be transmitted to an international audience, may both be seen as aggravating the offence; and in some legal systems the absence of any time limit on liability (in English law, for example, a new date of publication is established each time the same item is read online [Edwards and Waelde, 2009, 52]) adds a further element of risk.

While this may not seem at first glance to be a matter of great concern for the librarian who maintains a blog, in either a personal or an institutional capacity, the risk becomes considerably greater if that same blog permits readers to post their own unmoderated comments. Twitter, while it has the same characteristics of speed and internationality, is in some respects a less risky medium, since its limit of 140 characters per message may act as a natural form of restraint; but that same limit may also lead a twitterer to cut corners and, in doing so, to imply something that would not have been present in a longer statement.

Data protection issues must be considered with care. In each web-based service operated by a library, the likelihood is that data about its users will be collected – in the form of e-mail addresses, logon identifiers, cookies and other records of usage. Where the service involves a third-party host the risks, and thus the need to ensure that privacy can be maintained, are even greater. Edwards (Lex Ferenda, 2010) has identified the problems that can arise when the third party in question has very restrictive practices on access to the data it holds.

A third area of likely difficulty relates to copyright, intellectual property, and plagiarism. For example, the ease with which text and images can be cut and pasted into web-based library services may blind the blogger or mashup designer to the need to observe the necessary legal formalities. The manager of these services needs to be vigilant in ensuring that rights are observed, and must also have in place a suitable 'take-down' procedure for removing items that are challenged.

Guidance for the healthcare librarian

It should be clear from the foregoing that when we set out to use Web 2.0 applications we have to be aware of the possible dangers involved and will be well advised to undertake a realistic risk assessment. In the institutional environment this may be a formal organizational procedure that all staff have to observe, but even where it is not obligatory, the conscientious professional should be thinking critically about the possible pitfalls. This means not only being aware of the more obvious legal requirements, but also ensuring that the Web 2.0 users' conduct is consistent with the ethical standards expected of them.

We are able to draw on a number of codes of ethical practice from different countries. In some cases, codes framed specifically for healthcare information professionals are available (European Association for Health Information and Libraries, 2002; Medical Library Association, 2010), while in other countries the healthcare information profession relies on more general statements issued by parent bodies ([UK] Chartered Institute of Library and Information Professionals, 2009a, 2009b) or other authorities, as in the case of the Canadian Health Libraries Association/Association des bibliothèques de la santé du Canada, which relies on the Medical Library Association code just cited. It will quickly become apparent that none of these codes or the many others like them (IFLA, 2010) attempts to address issues arising specifically from activity on the internet, let alone from the use of Web 2.0 applications; but that is not a criticism. These codes lay down general standards that can and should be applied in all areas of the healthcare information professional's working life. It follows that, if a professional is charged with negligence by an aggrieved client, such as a library user, the ability to demonstrate that their actions were consistent with reasonable professional behaviour, as decreed by their fellow-professionals and defined in the relevant code, will form an important part of any defence.

Conclusion

Given the rapidly changing legal framework for regulation of the internet and the web, it is not realistic – and indeed might be dangerously misleading – for a chapter of this sort, written by a non-lawyer, to cite specific laws and rulings as a definitive statement of what is permissible or forbidden. The obvious caveat applies, that nothing here should be taken as authoritative legal advice. The reader who needs such advice must seek that from competent authorities with an up-to-date knowledge of the law, both nationally and internationally, as it affects internet use. It is, though, more realistic to offer guidance on good practice and the principles on which it is based; and for the reader who wishes to be as well prepared as possible by monitoring current thinking, draft legislation under discussion, court rulings or legal analysis, many sources of current awareness are available to a non-legally trained audience. Perhaps ironically but not surprisingly, a rich vein of material is to be found in the blogosphere and on other websites, and a short list of some useful sources that are regularly updated is provided at the end of this chapter.

It is rather too easy for a discussion of ethical and legal issues to sound negative and discouraging. We should, rather, heed the advice of Jing Jih Chin (Chin, 2010, 3), who, writing about doctors' attitudes to social networking, has observed that 'a knee-jerk reaction to reject any new technology or platform that appears to threaten professionalism risks rendering ... practitioners irrelevant'. The evidence to date is that few librarians, in healthcare or elsewhere, have yet been on the receiving end of legal actions because of their misuse of web applications, charged with a failure to maintain the necessary ethical standards. A sensible policy of vigilance is likely to ensure that this state of affairs continues.

Ethical and legal issues – bibliography and further reading

Bagnall, M. (2009) *Seeking Privacy in the Clouds* (blogpost), http://news.duke.edu/2009/10/osnprivacy.html.

Chaplin, C. (1964) *My Autobiography*, Bodley Head.

Chartered Institute of Library and Information Professionals (2009a) *Code of Professional Practice*, www.cilip.org.uk/get-involved/policy/ethics/pages/code.aspx.

Chartered Institute of Library and Information Professionals (2009b) *Ethical Principles for Library and Information Professionals*, www.cilip.org.uk/get-involved/policy/ethics/pages/principles.aspx.

Chin, J. J. (2010) Editorial – Medical Professionalism in the Internet Age, *Annals of the Academy of Medicine Singapore*, **39** (5), 1–3, www.annals.edu.sg/pdf/39VolNo5May2010/V39N5p345.pdf.

Edwards, L. and Waelde, C. (eds) (2009) *Law and the Internet*, 3rd edn, Hart Publishing.

European Association for Health Information and Libraries (2002) *Code of Ethics for EAHIL Members*, www.eahil.net/code_ethics.htm.

Healthcare Blogger Code of Ethics (2009) http://medbloggercode.com/the-code/.

IFLA (2010) *Professional Codes of Ethics for Librarians*, www.ifla.org/en/faife/professional-codes-of-ethics-for-librarians.

Kelly, B. (2010) A Deployment Strategy for Maximising the Impact of Institutional Use of Web 2.0. In Parkes, D. and Walton, G. (eds), *Web 2.0 and Libraries: impacts, technologies and trends*, Chandos Publishing.

Kevan, T. and McGrath, P. (2001) *E-mail, the Internet and the Law: essential knowledge for safer surfing*, EMIS Professional.

Legal Writing Prof Blog (2009) *The Liability Pitfalls of Twitter*, http://lawprofessors.typepad.com/legalwriting/2009/05/the-liability-pitfalls-of-twitter.html.

Lex Ferenda (2010) *Edwards: death and the web*, www.lexferenda.com/02062010/edwards-death-and-the-web/.

Medical Library Association (2010) *Code of Ethics for Health Sciences Librarianship*, www.mlanet.org/about/ethics.html.

Oppenheim, C. (2001) *The Legal and Regulatory Environment for Electronic Information*, 4th edn, Infonortics.

Ringmar, E. (2007) *A Blogger's Manifesto: free speech and censorship in the age of the internet*, Anthem Press, http://ia311024.us.archive.org/3/items/ABloggersManifestoFreeSpeechAndCensorshipInTheAgeOfTheInternet/ErikRingmarABloggersManifesto.pdf.

Rundle, A. and Conley, C. (2009) *Ethical Implications of Emerging Technologies: a survey*,

UNESCO, http://unesdoc.unesco.org/images/0014/001499/149992E.pdf.

Solove, D. J. (2007) *The Future of Reputation: gossip, rumor, and privacy on the internet*, Yale University Press.

Trushina, I. (2004) Freedom of Access: ethical dilemmas for internet librarians, *Electronic Library*, **22** (5), 416–21.

Zimmer, M. (2009) *Library 2.0, Access to Knowledge and Patron Privacy: avoiding a Faustian bargain*, http://michaelzimmer.org/files/Zimmer_Yale_L2.0_presentation.pdf.

Ethical and legal issues – useful blogs and wikis

EthicalLibrarian, http://ethicallibs.blogspot.com/.

HLWIKI Canada: Bloggers – Legal Aspects,
    http://hlwiki.slais.ubc.ca/index.php/Bloggers_-_Legal_aspects.

HLWIKI Canada: Ethics and the health librarian,
    http://hlwiki.slais.ubc.ca/index.php/Ethics_and_the_health_librarian.

HLWIKI Canada: Liability and the health librarian,
    http://hlwiki.slais.ubc.ca/index.php/Liability_of_health_librarians.

Information Ethicist, http:// infoethicist.blogspot.com/.

IPKat, http://ipkitten.blogspot.com/.

LibraryLaw Blog, http://blog.librarylaw.com/librarylaw/.

Michael Zimmer.org: Information ethics, new media, privacy, values in design,
    http://michaelzimmer.org/.

panGloss: a UK-based cyberlaw blog, http://blogscript.blogspot.com/.

WeblogTools Collection, 'Web Ethics' category,
    http://weblogtoolscollection.com/category/web-ethics/.

Website Law, www.website-law.co.uk/.

PART 3

Web applications in health information provision: some practical examples

CHAPTER 9

Web 2.0 in health libraries

Pip Divall

Introduction

Web 2.0 technologies are becoming increasingly important in healthcare (Randeree, 2009; Van De Belt et al., 2010). Health librarians and information professionals need to keep up to date with developments in technology and the latest in health information in order to support evidence-based healthcare (Sackett et al., 1996). In this chapter I will draw on specific examples of how health librarians make use of Web 2.0 technologies to enhance their work and support clinicians in their clinical practice, using my own experience as a Clinical Librarian at University Hospitals of Leicester (UHL) NHS Trust. I will present three case studies on different applications for Web 2.0 technology: the Clinical Librarian Blog; the UHL Writing Club wiki; and the Clinical Librarian Podcast; as well as the rationale for their use.

UHL NHS Trust is a large teaching hospital trust, with over 11,000 staff providing acute and secondary care to Leicester, Leicestershire and Rutland. There are three main hospital sites within the city: the Glenfield Hospital, Leicester General Hospital and the Leicester Royal Infirmary. UHL NHS Trust has two Trust-owned libraries, based at the Glenfield and Leicester General hospitals, and provides remote services to the Leicester Royal Infirmary, although there is a physical library there offering basic loan services to NHS staff.

The Clinical Librarian Service at UHL NHS Trust has been in place since its pilot in 2000, and has expanded over the years to three full-time Clinical Librarians (CLs) providing a service to most of the main clinical and corporate areas within the Trust. Two CLs support the clinical teams: Accident and Emergency; Anaesthesia; Cancer; Cardiorespiratory; Children's Services; Diabetes; Gastroenterology; Musculoskeletal; Renal and Transplant Services; Stroke; Surgery; and Women's, Perinatal and Sexual Health. The third CL supports corporate areas, including audit and infection control. This means that the CL maintains close contact with the teams, often attending ward rounds and case meetings so as to be best placed to understand the context of the question and the need for information, as well as acting as a prompt for the Trust staff to ask for a search of the evidence base to support their decisions.

Blogs and RSS feeds

Blogs, or weblogs, are online journals that can be used for many different purposes. They may be kept private, or be open and therefore used as a way of communicating with a wider audience. They may be written by a single author or by a group working collaboratively. Readers of the blog may also be able to comment on the posts and share their opinions and ideas.

RSS feeds (Really Simple Syndication or Rich Site Summary) are ways of pushing out newly published information from websites to a 'feed reader' so that users of the site may read what has been newly published to a site without visiting the site itself. They can cover any type of information that a website adds, and can be useful for sites that are updated regularly and that users may not have time to visit on a daily basis.

Blogs

Many libraries now use blogs and RSS to inform their users of new developments, for current awareness of journal contents and for general news items. The Health Library and Information Services Directory (http://hlisd.org) is run as a collaboration between the CILIP Health Libraries Group (HLG) and SHALL (Strategic Health Authority Library Leads) and allows NHS libraries wishing to use the facility to set up and push out RSS feeds, which then appear through the 'My Library' section of the NHS Evidence website (www.library.nhs.uk/mylibrary/default.aspx). However, constraints to this are finding the time to update the feed, and educating library users to make use of the service.

Since the advent of blogging, sites such as blogger.com have allowed users to create free blogs with custom names. Open source software with free hosting is a big consideration in health libraries, where there are strict controls over budgets and information technology.

Health information blogs can be a useful base for discussion of new resources and ideas. The blog run by a group of four health information professionals, Health Informaticist (http://healthinformaticist.wordpress.com), is one such blog where professional issues are discussed alongside new developments, changes in political focus and the art of blogging itself. For example, this blog contributes to Medlib's Round, where one blog summarizes noteworthy posts on a particular topic by the blogosphere (the blogging community) that have been submitted for the round.

Case study – Clinical Librarian blog

At UHL NHS Trust, the Clinical Librarians run a blog (http://clinicallibrarian.blogspot.com) (Figure 9.1) which is used primarily to discuss issues relating to the profession. Our blog began in November 2006, when I set it up, and has been running ever since. I set it up primarily as an experiment to see how it might work and to try out the new technology for ourselves. The aim is for the blog to be a hub for any

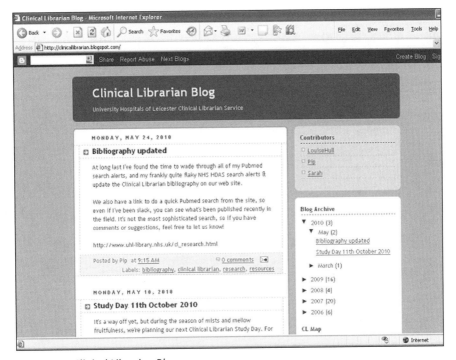

Figure 9.1 *Clinical Librarian Blog*

information that might interest or entertain our fellow Clinical Librarians, as well as to promote events that we run, such as the International Clinical Librarian Conference and various study days. While the blog does not generate a great deal of comment within the posts, we are able to track usage of the page using a free online visitor statistics tool (www.statcounter.com), which shows that readers come from as far afield as Iran and Australia. I check the statistics on a regular basis to see whether anyone is reading the blog and to remind myself that I should make more use of it. The average site-visit time is 2–3 minutes, so it appears we need snappy and punchy topics to hold the interest of our audience.

We aim to update the blog on a regular basis, but this can slip, due to other workloads. Our experience is that blogging is a task that you have to set for yourself to do on a regular basis so as to maintain readership, and generating comment can be difficult. It has also been difficult to convince my fellow CLs to take part in authoring posts, so the burden of thinking up topics is not always shared.

The blog also has a link to a 'map of Clinical Librarians', created using Google maps (Figure 9.2). The pins on the map are placed by CLs themselves, so that a picture of where they are operating in the UK and beyond is emerging. Not all of the CLs we are aware of are represented on the map as yet, and it would be interesting to see if we are able to expand to those working under different job titles in the USA as well. The highest concentration of CLs on the map is in the north of England, which fits with

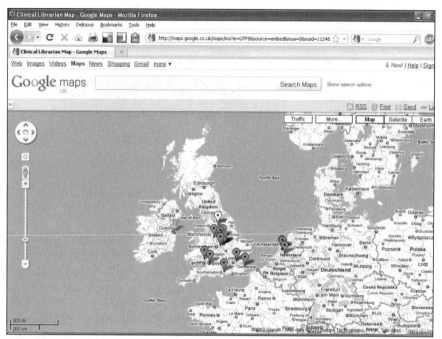

Figure 9.2 *Clinical Librarian Map*

the picture we have of employed CLs who registered to have their contact details on our website. However, many CLs we know of in the UK have not yet taken up the map idea. Several of our colleagues in the Netherlands have placed their pins on the map, showing our international links.

RSS feeds

Using a feed reader, such as Google Reader (www.google.com/reader) or Bloglines (www.bloglines.com), it is possible to set up all your RSS feeds for viewing in one place. Bloglines announced in September 2010 that it was to close on 1 October 2010, citing Twitter as a major cause of a decline in RSS aggregator usage, and this decline and a change in its owners' business focus are the main factors in this decision. However, I still find RSS feeds incredibly useful in keeping up to date, and I transferred my feeds from Bloglines to Google Reader in 2007.

Finding blogs with RSS feeds for potential use is simple, by looking out for the orange RSS symbol or by using aggregators, such as www.medworm.com, or the internal search functionality of the feed reader you choose to use. The 'blogosphere' is doubling in size every six months, with over 50 million blogs now online (McLean, Richards and Wardman, 2007). Using a search facility such as MedWorm allows the user to be more circumspect in selecting appropriate blogs to follow.

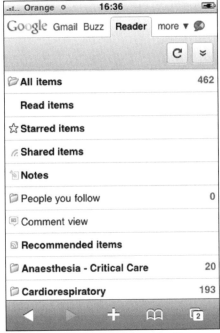

Figure 9.3 *Google Reader on the iPhone*

RSS feeds can be useful for horizon scanning and keeping up to date on new publications from any number of sources. The NHS Evidence Specialist Collections (www.evidence.nhs.uk/aboutus/Pages/ Listofspecialistcollections.aspx) provides RSS feeds of new additions to the collections, which are generally new publications from a variety of accredited health resources, including NICE (the National Institute for Health and Clinical Excellence). Feeds can also be used to keep up to date on a particular topic or search question, through using sites such as hubmed.org, which is an interface for PubMed and automatically searches on a daily basis for your search string. Clinical staff with particular research interests can be supported in setting up their own feeds for topic areas, or the health librarian can look out for relevant articles on their behalf. Library staff can also assist clinicians in finding suitable RSS feeds and blogrolls (lists of blogs).

RSS feeds have been incredibly useful to me in allowing me to keep up with new publications in the clinical areas that I support. I have been able to find out when studies are published that the clinicians I work with are interested in reading, and then deliver the documents directly to the ward round, where previously I might have had to scan journal contents pages either electronically or by hand. Time saving is the major advantage of using RSS feeds, as all your favourite web pages can be checked together on the one site. The blogosphere has lamented the loss of Bloglines, and many feel that RSS feeds still have a lot to contribute to Web 2.0.

RSS feed reader applications are now available for Android and iPhones (Figure 9.3) as paid-for and free applications, and many feed readers are available in mobile versions for PDAs and internet-enabled mobile phones, allowing users to keep up to date on the move.

Wikis

From the Hawaiian 'to hurry' or 'quick', the word 'wiki' has also become a recursive acronym, standing for 'what I know is'. Wikis are Web 2.0 applications that allow users to share information and collaborate online and enable them to edit the content of a website (Bastida, McGrath and Maude, 2010). Wiki sites are very useful as collaborative websites, using the functionality of shared authorship to build group sites. As they are open source software, some health libraries even use wikis as their main web presence rather than have an externally hosted website.

Case study: UHL Writing Club

Many hospital Trusts and clinical teams working in Trusts run their own journal clubs. These can be either formal or informal groups getting together on a regular basis to read and critique writing on current clinical topics, or to answer particular research questions using the best available evidence. The Writing Club is based on this model, and we gather together any interested parties on a quarterly basis to discuss a topic related to writing and also offer a clinic for any writing-related queries at the end of each session. UHL NHS Trust set up a Writing Club in 2009 and all the sessions we have held to date have been well attended by junior doctors, nurses, physiotherapists and medical students.

The impetus for the Writing Club came from the CLs, as I in particular wanted more help and advice on how to write for publication and had struggled to find any formal courses available. We also found that a lot of requests for information on how to write were coming from junior doctors within the Trust, as the pressure mounted up on them to publish case studies and reports.

We set up a wiki site (http://uhlwritingclub.pbworks.com) which is used to host slides from presentations that have been given at past sessions, as well as related links, useful articles (copyright permitting) and discussion of topics (Figure 9.4). The Club and wiki site are in their infancy, but all people attending the group are given authoring rights for the site when they give the organizers their e-mail addresses. Once a user has registered to become a writer on the site, they are authorized by the wiki owner and able to set up an account. There is no moderation by the administrator of the wiki, editors of the site are free to put up information, and the administrator can see what changes have been made. Further features and more administrative controls are available if a paid for subscription is purchased rather than the basic free subscription.

Direct upload to the wiki site means that it can be updated at any time, from any workstation, and allows the pages to be dynamic. There is no need to have special web-authoring software to make changes to the content, or to go through any protocol for uploading the content. It is also possible to subscribe to the wiki as an RSS feed and thus be notified by that means of any changes to the content. It is possible to comment on the pages or to make changes to the content of any author, but the owner of the site retains the administration right to allow the changes to take place.

The wiki site is used to promote sessions of the Writing Club, as a repository for presentations made so far and as a resource library for referencing help, statistics and opportunities for research. There are also links to local e-learning packages that should enable users to understand the process of writing up a research paper more thoroughly and therefore assist in their goal of publishing a paper. The e-learning packages cover

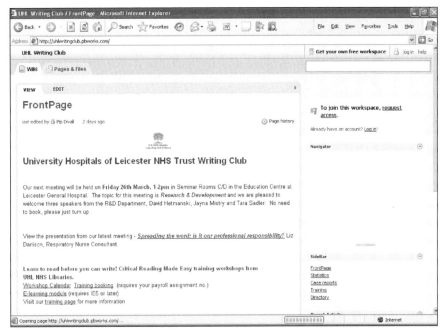

Figure 9.4 *UHL Writing Club Wiki*

aspects of literature searching in the biomedical databases and how to go about critically appraising published scientific papers.

We are currently investigating how we may be able to measure the impact of the Writing Club so as to find out if the participants have benefited from attendance and if the number of articles being published by staff at UHL NHS Trust has increased since the establishment of the Club. Topics covered by the Club so far have been writing case reports; basic statistics; how to obtain ethical approval for research projects; and using reference management software.

Podcasts

Podcasts are audio or video content created for the potential audience to download and listen to or watch wherever or whenever they choose to do so. Educational aspects of podcasts include listening to lectures; watching demonstrations of particular techniques; or listening to groups of experts discussing topics of interest. Podcasts also use RSS feed technology and are built into web browsers such as Internet Explorer 7 and Mozilla Firefox.

Several health resources now utilize podcasts to deliver information. For example, the Cochrane Library uses them for new systematic reviews (www.thecochranelibrary. com). The use of podcasts is now becoming a far wider phenomenon as information providers acquire the means to upload content in different media. Podcasts have the advantage of offering learning in a style that may suit individuals better than simply reading material in print (Kamel Boulos, Maramba and Wheeler, 2006).

Authors submitting to journals are now also encouraged to upload video content to supplement written articles.

Case study: Building the Brazilian Bridge project podcast

In 2008, the UHL NHS Trust Clinical Librarians were invited to take part in the Building the Brazilian Bridge project, which was begun by the Department of Information Science, Loughborough University, and the Department of Orthopaedic Surgery in PUC-Campinas, Brazil (Marão Beraquet, Harrison and Ciol, 2009). Our involvement as CLs was in making a podcast discussing our roles as CLs, for broadcast to CLs just starting out in their careers in South America (Harrison, 2008, www-staff.lboro.ac.uk/~lsjr1/index.htm). This was a very useful experience for us as well, as we are often asked to talk about our service, and we are now able to direct other health information professionals to the podcast for a quick overview of how we work. However, this is something that will need updating as the service evolves to suit the needs of the organization where we work. The podcast was broadcast in a workshop to a group of interested Brazilian librarians who were considering whether to participate in a CL pilot project and led to a project that was successfully completed. The aim was to show how the CL service works in the UK and give the Brazilian librarians an idea of how they might be able to implement the model in their own setting.

Twitter

Twitter.com, the microblogging site in which updates or 'tweets' can be no more than 140 characters long, has great potential for evidence-based healthcare. Many health sites have channels, including the *HSJ* (*Health Service Journal*) and the NHS Evidence Specialist Collections. The usefulness of Twitter is similar to that of RSS feeds, in that new publications or developments may get tweeted before they become widely available, and so CLs are able to deliver the documents to customers in a timely way. Two of the three CLs at UHL NHS Trust are currently making use of Twitter, and so far we have found it to be extremely helpful. As it was a restricted site by the Trust Information Management Team, a formal application to be excepted from the ban was necessary and had to be authorized by a senior manager. Since our access has been granted, the CLs have been using Twitter as an adjunct to their RSS feeds, and keeping up to date with newly published information by following people and organizations working in the clinical areas we support. This has been extremely useful in enabling us to update our clinical teams with information they may find useful as it becomes available. I have been able to pass on NICE Guidance on stroke care to the multidisciplinary team I work with via a link from Twitter, and I have also been able to pass information on smoking cessation statistics to a consultant respiratory intensivist whom I know to have a particular interest in the topic. This has definitely been appreciated by the teams I work with, who do not have time to monitor the sources that I am able to access.

Twitter was also used at the conferences we attended during 2010. At the European Association for Health Information and Libraries (EAHIL) Conference in Lisbon, Portugal (www.eahil2010.org), a dedicated group of health information professionals were tweeting their thoughts on the presentations as they occurred. Similarly, at the Health Libraries Group branch of CILIP's (www.cilip.org.uk/hlg) conference in 2010, delegates tweeted their impressions of the presentations they attended using the hashtag #hlg2010, which meant that tweets relating to the conference could be found easily by searching, or by using the conference 'twub' (http://twubs.com/hlg2010), which is a way of saving the tweets on a particular topic.

There can be significant personal and professional overlap in using Twitter, so it may be useful to consider separating out accounts for personal and professional use if you want to target a particular group of followers with your tweets.

Barriers to Web 2.0 in healthcare

Some librarians working in the NHS have found that new developments in information technology can be difficult to implement in a local setting. Due to the sensitive nature of some of the information that is available via NHS workstations, Trust information technology departments can be reluctant to allow access to Web 2.0 and social networking sites. Some NHS PCs have access to patient booking systems and sensitive personal data, so the integrity of networks is important. The fluid nature of these sites, and the crossover between personal and professional use can also be an issue. It may be that librarians and information professionals working in healthcare need to demonstrate the potential value of these sites and of Web 2.0 as a whole in order to gain regular access.

Another potential worry is somehow getting things wrong and starting a project that may not work out the way you had hoped. The ease of using Web 2.0 technologies means that it is simple to set up sites and blogs and try them out, without too much fear of it not working out. Giving something a go and failing does not mean you have not learned from the process. Some sites will make changes or begin to charge for a service, and this can mean that a lot of hard work could disappear, so it is best to check the robustness of a service before you start to use it. As with the demise of Bloglines, it does not always follow that being owned by a large company will protect a particular service from being cancelled or superseded. Many sites will allow you to export files or subscriptions to another service, or to a back-up file on your PC. Making sure that you actually use a service should mean that you will be apprised of any changes that may affect you. Things can change quickly in Web 2.0!

Conclusion

The experience of using Web 2.0 technologies as a CL at UHL NHS Trust has been mostly positive. We have tried out blogs and RSS feeds and found them to be useful. If I were starting out again, I would try to make the blog more collaborative than it currently is, but the beauty of Web 2.0 means that I am able to change my approach when I choose to. I did change RSS feed readers from Bloglines to Google Reader when I discovered that I preferred the style of Google Reader; it was not difficult to transfer my subscriptions. The main lesson I have drawn from my experience of Web 2.0 technologies in my work is that experimentation doesn't hurt and usually costs nothing but time.

Web 2.0 technologies are appealing to the new generation of healthcare professionals, who have grown up with social networking and collaborative websites. In terms of information literacy, some of the Web 2.0 methods may seem less daunting to use than more traditional methods. As our core customers begin to use Web 2.0 applications more in their day-to-day lives, they will become more competent and confident in making these useful in their work also.

Web 2.0 is still a developing area within healthcare librarianship, and new applications for the available resources are being found all the time. The experience of UHL NHS Trust is that it is a good idea to at least attempt to make use of the resources available in order to understand whether they can be used to help clinicians, other information professionals and the authors of a wiki, blog or RSS feed.

References and further reading

Bastida, R., McGrath, I. and Maude, P. (2010) Wiki Use in Mental Health Practice: recognizing potential use of collaborative technology, *International Journal of Mental Health Nursing*, **19** (2), 142–8.

Divall, P., Sutton, S. and Ward, L. (2007) Pharm-Assist: using personal digital assistants (PDAs) to assist in pharmacy decisions, *Journal of the European Association for Health Information and Libraries*, **3** (4), 24–30.

Harrison, J. (2008) *Clinical Librarianship - Building the Brazilian Bridge Project Introduction podcast*, http://www-staff.lboro.ac.uk/~lsjr1/CLIP%201.wmv.

Honeybourne, C., Ward, L., Sutton, S. A., Powell, R. and Divall, P. (2007) *Personal Digital Assistants for Foundation Doctors: handheld knowledge in the clinical setting*, University of Leicester, unpublished study.

Kamel Boulos, M. N., Maramba, I. and Wheeler, S. (2006) Wikis, Blogs and Podcasts: a new generation of web-based tools for virtual collaborative clinical practice and education, *BMC Medical Education*, **6**, 41.

Marão Beraquet, V.S., Harrison, J. and Ciol, R. (2009) Breaching the library walls in Brazil - clinical librarianship in Celso Pierro Hospital: a pilot study. In: *Positioning the Profession: the Tenth International Congress on Medical Librarianship*, Brisbane, Australia, (1–5), August 31–September 4, 2009, http://espace.library.uq.edu.au/view/UQ:179729.

McLean, R., Richards, B. H. and Wardman, J. I. (2007) The Effect of Web 2.0 on the Future of Medical Practice and Education: Darwikian evolution or folksonomic revolution? *The Medical Journal of Australia*, **187** (3), 174–7.

Randeree, E. (2009) Exploring Technology Impacts of Healthcare 2.0 Initiatives, *Telemedicine Journal and E-health*, **15** (3), 255–60.

Sackett, D. L., Rosenberg, W. M., Gray, J. A., Haynes, R. B. and Richardson, W. S. (1996) Evidence Based Medicine: what it is and what it isn't, *BMJ*, **312** (7023), 71.

Stokes, T., Shaw, E. J., Camosso-Stefinovic, J., Powell, R., Ward, L., Rimmington, P., Seare, N. and Baker, R. (2006) *The Role of Portable Electronic Technologies in Reducing the Risk of Adverse Events Following Patient Handovers: systematic review*, University Hospitals of Leicester NHS Trust, unpublished study.

Van De Belt, T. H., Engelen, L. J., Berben, S. A. and Schoonhoven, L. (2010) Definition of Health 2.0 and Medicine 2.0: a systematic review, *Journal of Medical Internet Research*, **12** (2), e18.

CHAPTER 10

RSS (Really Simple Syndication): helping faculty and residents stay up to date

Thane Chambers, Dale Storie and Sandy Campbell

Introduction

It is imperative that clinicians and researchers in the health sciences stay current with advances in their fields. Many find themselves pressed for time and struggle with the volume of information available to them (Davies, 2007; Wallis, 2006). RSS (Really Simple Syndication) offers a relatively simple approach to managing the flow of new information that is published on the web. This chapter presents an overview of RSS and a case study of teaching RSS to health sciences faculty and medical residents.

What is RSS?

RSS is a web-based syndication format that allows information feeds from multiple websites to be aggregated into one place. Typically, the information from an RSS feed is sent directly to a user's desktop or web browser via a feed reader (also known as an aggregator), so that whenever a website is updated the user receives the new information automatically.

From a technology perspective, RSS is an XML-based format which is fairly simple for information services and content providers to produce and for consumers to use. It is commonly used to subscribe to blogs and podcasts, as well as to generate dynamic web content (e.g. personalized home pages such as iGoogle). RSS originated in the late 1990s but did not become popular until the rise of Web 2.0 in the mid 2000s.

RSS in library and information services

Many librarians have identified RSS as a beneficial technology for current awareness. Librarians have traditionally been involved with the provision of current awareness services such as selective dissemination of information (SDI). These services have taken a variety of forms, from creating specialized publications that identify new literature to setting up electronic database alerts (Anderson, 1998; Shultz and De Groote, 2003). RSS feeds are perceived as being especially valuable for academics and professionals because they make use of a single interface (the feed reader) to manage information from new media such as websites and blogs, as well as from traditional information sources such as scholarly journals (Anderson, 2006; Cooke, 2006; Giustini, 2006).

Much of the journal literature about RSS is purely descriptive, focusing on what the technology is and how it can be used in libraries or information services (Cohen, 2008; Holvoet, 2006; Tennant, 2003). In implementation, RSS has been used to promote new resources, deliver library news, and provide database alerts (Armstrong, 2007; Blansit, 2006; Corrado and Moulaison, 2006). Health sciences librarians have discussed the technology explicitly as a means of providing current awareness services to clients (Broun, 2004; Cooke, 2006; Estabrook, 2005; Johnson, Osmond and Holz, 2009; Neilson, 2008).

However, as Neilson (2008) points out, little literature exists that evaluates end-user uptake of RSS-based library and information services. Within the broader population, data suggest that only a minority of web-connected individuals use RSS feeds. Although the orange RSS button is ubiquitous on the web, a number of surveys on the use of online media show that, overall, fewer than 15% of internet users actually use RSS feeds. According to surveys of regular internet users, the rate of adoption has gone from 5% in 2005 to between 8% and 12% in 2008 (De Rosa and OCLC, 2005; Pew Research Center for People and the Press, 2008). Furthermore, a Forrester Research report (Katz et al., 2008) which found very little interest in RSS from non-users suggests that adoption may have already peaked.

This low rate of adoption and potential barriers for users have been acknowledged and discussed in several evaluative articles. At the National Cancer Institute, Broun (2004) realized that few clients were using RSS and opted to provide a service that compiled RSS feeds from various sources into an e-mail digest. Neilson (2008, 57–67), meanwhile, heavily promoted an RSS service at the Health Quality Council, and although many of her users expressed interest, many still found that e-mail fitted into their workflow better. For many users, it appears that any potential advantage of using RSS does not necessarily outweigh the advantages of familiar technologies such as listservs and e-mail alerts.

Furthermore, there is emerging recognition that RSS may not be as straightforward as many early adopters had expected. Fletcher (2009) discusses potential problems that librarians may encounter when teaching users about RSS, such as content authentication and inconsistent feed data. Johnson et al. (2009), arguing that managing RSS journal updates from multiple providers can 'frustrate and overwhelm even the savviest user' (52), introduced a current awareness service that attempted to address technological hurdles by pre-bundling journal feeds by subject for researchers to upload into their aggregator. Miles (2009) has suggested that RSS is still invaluable as an invisible background technology, regardless of whether end-users adopt it.

The library literature indicates that among faculty and professionals there is a demand for training (Akers, Martin and Summey, 2000; Quigley, Church and Peterson, 2001; Mackenzie and Makin, 2003), yet only a few articles have discussed teaching end-users about RSS (Fletcher, 2009; Neilson, 2008). RSS may be relatively easy to use and there are plenty of online tutorials to assist new users, but finding the time to learn the details of a new technology is difficult, especially when its benefits may not be immediately evident. The following case study illustrates the role that formal instruction can play in learning about RSS, and provides some context for understanding the experience of end-users.

Case study: University of Alberta John W. Scott Health Sciences Library
Context

The John W. Scott Health Sciences Library (Scott Library) at the University of Alberta in Edmonton, Alberta, Canada, serves five health sciences faculties: Faculty of Medicine and Dentistry, Faculty of Pharmacy and Pharmaceutical Sciences, Faculty of Rehabilitation Medicine, Faculty of Nursing and the School of Public Health. These faculties offer undergraduate and graduate education. The Faculty of Medicine and Dentistry also supports a large medical resident training programme. All of the faculties have robust research programmes. The research and teaching programme is closely integrated with the local hospitals, including the University of Alberta Hospital, which is a teaching hospital adjacent to the campus. The Scott Library is physically connected to the hospital and academic buildings.

Through anecdotal evidence, the librarians at the Scott Library became aware of both the challenges faced by faculty and residents in managing new information and the fact that few of the faculty and residents were using RSS feeds. The librarians speculated that the time needed to learn RSS was a barrier to its use.

Initial survey

To test these suppositions and to determine the level of interest in RSS, health sciences faculty members and medical residents were invited to take part in an online survey. One hundred and sixty-four people responded to the survey. The results revealed a high interest in RSS feeds, but relatively low use of and familiarity with them. Of the respondents, 52.4% had never heard of RSS feeds, while 41.4% had some awareness or had tried to use them. Only 6.1% (ten people) were checking RSS feeds on a regular basis (either daily, weekly or monthly).

The most prevalent themes in the comments indicated that lack of time, lack of knowledge and fear of being overwhelmed by information were barriers to faculty and residents' use of RSS technology.

Among the few comments related to benefits, the most common themes related to 'time savings' and 'keeping current'. Overall, however, respondents were very interested in learning more about RSS, with 89.9% indicating that they were interested in attending an instructional session. This encouraged the research team to proceed with offering classes designed to introduce faculty and students to RSS.

Instruction session

Respondents who had indicated an interest in attending a session on RSS were invited to participate in one of four classes. These classes were also available to people in the original target group who had not responded to the survey. Four classes entitled 'Current awareness using RSS feeds' were offered over two months. Classes were offered on various weekdays and at varying times of the day. They were advertised on the Library's homepage, on posters and flyers handed out at the desk and through e-mail to people who had expressed an interest.

Participants in the classes were surveyed before the class. The responses to this survey were similar to those of the broader survey: 60.9% had never heard of RSS, 34.8% were aware of RSS feeds but had not tried them and 4.3% had set up feeds but weren't checking them or had had problems. None of the 23 people who attended the classes were using RSS feeds regularly.

The participants in the class were also asked what kinds of content they wanted to receive through RSS feeds. Their replies indicated that 90.9% wanted to receive new professional or academic articles in their fields, 45% wanted to be alerted when a particular article was cited, 31.8% wanted to receive personal current-interest information such as weather, news, sports or stock market information, 18.2% wanted alerts when something was posted to a blog or listserv or when there was a change to a website. All of these topics were covered during the instructional sessions.

Each of the four classes was conducted in a computer lab to allow hands-on learning. Drawing from research that suggests that professional development training is successful when it incorporates active learning components (Armstrong and Barsion, 2006, 483–8; Knox, 2003, 141–5), the instructors encouraged participants to follow along with them during the class. After a brief introduction, a librarian led the class through the process of signing up for RSS feeds from several different kinds of services. These included a Medline search alert, a news alert, a professional journal table-of-contents alert and a citation alert. The instructor demonstrated Google Reader as an example of a web-based RSS reader and Internet Explorer as an example of a browser-based reader.

Participants were given a detailed handout that described the procedures for the class so that they could follow along and make notes. Two additional librarians were available during each class to work individually with participants and ensure that they were able to accomplish each step. By the end of the classes, all attendees had actively participated in creating an account with an RSS aggregator and had subscribed to several feeds.

Following the classes, participants completed an evaluative questionnaire which asked whether they had found the class to be useful, whether their learning goals had been met, and if they expected to use RSS feeds in the future. All 23 participants in the classes returned the questionnaire, but not all answered every question. Of those who answered (n=22), 100% found the session 'useful' or 'sort of useful', and 100% (n=23) said they would recommend it to a friend.

Satisfaction with the session was also reflected in such comments as:

- 'I need something and this is *great*!'
- 'Will definitely use them to capture more current awareness/update info than I'm covering now.'

Nine of the 23 comments referred to the value of the hands-on part of the class.

Follow-up survey

Approximately two months after the last instructional session, an invitation was e-mailed to each class participant, asking them to complete a survey which explored their current activities with RSS feeds. The survey was administered electronically through Survey Monkey.

Fifteen participants responded to the survey. Participants could respond in more than one category. The responses showed that 66.7% had become more aware of RSS feeds; 46.7% had talked with someone about RSS feeds; 53.3% had recommended RSS feeds to someone else; 46.7% had used their RSS feed to receive information. While 46.7% had done nothing with their RSS feeds, 6.7% had set up feeds but were not using them, while 20.0% were getting too much information. No one had tried unsuccessfully to set up another feed.

Participants were also given an opportunity to comment on their use of RSS feeds. Several themes emerged regarding barriers to use. These were expressed in various ways, such as:

- 'I have not had time to fully implement it.'
- 'Not yet [implemented], due to time constraints/priorities.'

Several also expressed getting too much information, indicating that they needed to fine-tune their use through better organization and filtering. For example:

- 'A bit overwhelming having so much information coming in every day.'
- 'Still trying to figure out the best way to organize.'
- 'It can take a while to get your RSS feed to perform like you want it to.'

One person also commented that 'some of the sites I use regularly don't offer RSS feeds'. However, many comments also reflected themes of success with RSS feeds. The most prominent were related to the ease of keeping up to date and the ability to control the flow of information:

- 'I was able to keep up to date on new papers.'
- 'I can control what I want to see.'
- 'You don't have to go looking for information.'

When participants were asked how RSS compared to e-mail alerts, responses were varied. Some preferred e-mail because it was more active and less easy to forget, while others preferred having journal alerts separated from e-mail. As one respondent commented, 'they are both similar, it is just choosing what works best for you'.

Beyond the effect on participants, there was also an observable multiplier effect that fanned out from the instruction sessions. One of the participants noted: 'I have done nothing personally with RSS feeds, but have passed on the benefit to others working in my research group.' Participants also referred several people to the library for information about RSS feeds. Content from the session has also been used in a training programme for rural doctors.

Lessons learned and best practices

From this case study we can draw several conclusions. First, while RSS is fairly simple technology, some people just do not have the time, inclination or resources to learn it on their own. Therefore these people benefit from receiving instruction in a more formal and structured setting, rather than trying to make time to work through online tutorials or read instructions. Participants in the class appreciated the hands-on learning and had many questions that the librarian-instructors could answer on the spot. Almost half of the classroom participants moved from non-use of RSS feeds to continued use of RSS feeds and were finding some efficiencies in using them.

Second, many participants still had questions and problems. The need for more knowledge may be mitigated with further use, but a series of laddered sessions on RSS may be another option for libraries. Users could have an introductory session, have an opportunity to explore using RSS on their own, and then return for a follow-up session where questions or problems could be addressed.

Third, it is obvious that RSS is not a cure-all for helping this population to control the flow of information. Some people were clearly getting too much information and others found little benefit over existing e-mail alerts. Further study could be done to determine if users need more training to solve the overload problem or if it is the result of RSS feeds not allowing users to fine-tune the content that they receive.

Finally, further research needs to be done to determine whether or not the changes in behaviour observed in participants in this study are long lasting. Ideally, participants who adopted RSS feeds would be resurveyed to determine whether or not their behavioural changes were long lasting and if they had found ways to make efficient use of RSS feeds.

Conclusion

As a fairly simple technology, RSS offers great potential for library and information services. However, many users are unfamiliar with it, do not perceive its benefits, and are not willing to learn it on their own. The case study indicates that teaching RSS to health sciences faculty and medical residents helps to mitigate some of these factors, leading to increased awareness and use of RSS in the short term. However, RSS does not solve problems of information overload and some users still prefer e-mail for staying up to date.

References

Akers, C., Martin, N. and Summey, T. (2000) Teaching the Teachers: library instruction through professional development courses, *Research Strategies*, **17** (2/3), 215–21.

Anderson, B. (2006) Keeping Up: SDI to RSS, *Behavioral and Social Sciences Librarian*, **24** (2), 113–17.

Anderson, C. (1998) Proactive Reference, *Reference and User Services Quarterly*, **38** (2), 139–40.

Armstrong, E. G. and Barsion, S. J. (2006) Using an Outcomes-logic-model Approach To Evaluate a Faculty Development Program for Medical Educators, *Academic Medicine: Journal of the Association of American Medical Colleges*, **81** (5), 483–8.

Armstrong, K. (2007) Using RSS Feeds to Alert Users to Electronic Resources, *The Serials Librarian*, **53** (3), 183–91.

Blansit, B. D. (2006) Using RSS to Publish Library News and Information, *Journal of Electronic Resources in Medical Libraries*, **3** (1), 97–104.

Broun, K. (2004) New Dog, Old Trick: alerts for RSS feeds, *Library Journal; Summer Net Connect*, **18**, 20.

Cohen, S. (2008) The Power of RSS: instant information updating based on quality searches, *MultiMedia and Internet@Schools*, **15** (1), 15–17.

Cooke, C. A. (2006) Current Awareness in the New Millennium: RSS, *Medical Reference Services Quarterly*, **25** (1), 59–69.

Corrado, E. M. and Moulaison, H. L. (2006) Integrating RSS Feeds of New Books into the Campus Course Management System, *Computers in Libraries*, **26** (9), 6, 9, 61–2, 64.

Davies, K. (2007) The Information-seeking Behaviour of Doctors: a review of the evidence, *Health Information and Libraries Journal*, **24** (2), 78–94.

De Rosa, C. and OCLC (2005) *Perceptions of Libraries and Information Resources: a report to the OCLC membership*, OCLC.

Estabrook, A. D. (2005) Leveraging Real Simple Syndication for Current Awareness, *Journal of Hospital Librarianship*, **5** (3), 83–92.

Fletcher, A. M. (2009) Free-range RSS Feeds and Farm-raised Journals: WHAT to expect when using RSS as a TOC service, *Medical Reference Services Quarterly*, **28** (2), 172–9.

Giustini, D. (2006) How Web 2.0 Is Changing Medicine, *BMJ*, **333** (7582), 1283–4.

Holvoet, K. (2006) What Is RSS and How Can Libraries Use It to Improve Patron Service? *Library Hi Tech News*, **23** (8), 32–3.

Johnson, S. M., Osmond, A. and Holz, R. (2009) Developing a Current Awareness Service Using Really Simple Syndication (RSS), *Journal of the Medical Library Association: JMLA*, **97** (1), 52–4.

Katz, J. M., Overby, C. S., Owyang, J. K., Cummings, T. and Murphy, E. (2008) *What's Holding RSS Back? Consumers still don't understand this really simple technology*, Forrester Research, 47150.

Knox, A. B. (2003) Building on abilities, *Journal of Continuing Education in the Health Professions*, **23** (3), 141–5.

Mackenzie, A. and Makin, L. (2003) Beyond Student Instruction: information skills for staff, *New Review of Academic Librarianship*, **9**, 113–30.

Miles, A. (2009) RIP RSS: reviving innovative programs through really savvy services, *Journal of Hospital Librarianship*, **9** (4), 425–32.

Neilson, C. (2008) Current Awareness on a Shoe String: RSS at the HQC, *Internet Reference Services Quarterly*, **13** (1), 57–67.

Pew Research Center for People and the Press (2008) *Online and Digital News: key news audiences now blend online and traditional sources*, http://people-press.org/report/?pageid=1354.

Quigley, B. D., Church, G. M. and Peterson, A. (2001) Defining the Need for Information Technology Instruction among Science Faculty, *Science and Technology Libraries*, **20** (1), 5–42.

Shultz, M. and De Groote, S. L. (2003) MEDLINE SDI Services: how do they compare? *Journal of the Medical Library Association*, **91** (4), 460–7.

Tennant, R. (2003) Feed Your Head: keeping up by using RSS, *Library Journal (1976)*, **128** (9), 30.

Wallis, L. C. (2006) Information-seeking Behaviour of Faculty in One School of Public Health, *Journal of the Medical Library Association: JMLA*, **94** (4), 442–7.

CHAPTER 11

Using mashups in health information provision

Jukka Englund

Introduction

Scholarly publications are the end product of research work. In most cases the budgets of research groups rely on the productivity of group members: how many articles have been published and what are the Impact Factors of the journals? Thus, scholars strive for maximum visibility and impression in their publishing efforts.

Terkko – Meilahti Campus Library (formerly: Terkko – National Library of Health Sciences, Finland), now part of the Helsinki University Library, has done pioneering work to highlight scholarly publications in medicine and health sciences at faculty, university and national level in Finland through innovative library services.

The Library is using the latest technologies to disseminate information about research done in Finland. This case study presents some of the key services that the Library is offering so as to increase the global visibility and substance of Finnish medical research, and the Web 2.0 tools that are offered to library customers.

Past

Virtual Journal of Helsinki Medical Research (VJHMR)[1] was a monthly multi-journal compilation of the latest research at the University of Helsinki. It was published from 2000 until 2005. At that time, the publication provided a good overview of the scholarly publishing of the faculty. It had a major influence on the development of comparable services, for example Lund University, Sweden, published Lund Virtual Medical Journal from 2002 until 2007 (now Lund Medical Faculty Monthly).[2]

Technology

A Web 2.0. tool, RSS technology,[3] prepared the way for more rapid and automatic alerting of new articles. An RSS web feed is a data format used with frequently updated content, such as the bibliographical data on scientific articles published in scholarly journals. FeedNavigator,[4] a free web-feed aggregator made in Terkko, started as a medical and health sciences entity, but today it is a genuine multi-disciplinary alerting service. FeedNavigator downloads some 6000 feeds from journals, news services and blogs and also offers sophisticated tools that enable end-users to customize the interface. In addition, FeedNavigator downloads 600+ feeds of the latest articles published by Finnish scholars from the PubMed[5,6] database. These feeds are the backbone of the Scholar Chart mashup.

Present
Scholar Chart

Who is the Helsinki University medical scholar who has put out the most articles during the past 365 days? What are the average Impact Factors of these publications? In which journals are Finnish medical scholars publishing their work? And who is at the top of the Terkko Factor list this week? Scholar Chart,[7] a mashup made in Terkko, combines FeedNavigator RSS feeds, Impact Factors (IF), SCImago Journal Ranks (SJR) and the OpenCalais web service tag clouds in a highly unique way. A mashup is a web application that combines data from more than one source into a single integrated service. Scholar Chart lists some 620 Finnish medical scholars (from five medical universities and selected research institutions) and their article publications in real time.

The following set of values are represented: the absolute number of publications, the mean value of journals' (in which the scholar has published) Impact Factors, the mean value of journals' (in which the scholar has published) SCImago Journal Ranks and Terkko Factor (square root [average Impact Factor × average SJR] × number of publications). The lists can be sorted by all of these fields. The data are provided for the last 12 and 36 months.

Impact Factors

Journal Citation Reports® (JCR)[8] is a database from Thomson Reuters that provides quantitative tools for ranking, evaluating and comparing journals. To give an example of the tools, the Impact Factor (IF) helps to measure research influence and impact at the journal and category levels and shows the relationship between citing and cited journals.

SCImago Journal Ranks (SJR)

The SJR is an indicator that expresses the number of connections that a journal receives through the citation of its documents divided between the total of documents published in the year selected by the publication, weighted according to the number of incoming and outgoing connections of the sources. The SCImago Journal and Country Rank[9] is a portal that includes the journals and country scientific indicators developed from the information contained in the Scopus database.

Terkko Factor

Terkko Factor, listed exclusively on the Scholar Chart website, is a combination of the absolute number of publications and the Impact Factors and SCImago Journal Ranks of the journals of these publications.

OpenCalais tag clouds

A tag cloud, which depicts keywords extracted automatically from the titles and abstracts of articles by OpenCalais web service (Thomson Reuters), is provided for the whole of Finland and for each of the universities and institutions. It is thus an outstanding and transparent tool for quickly gaining an overview of what research topics are hot in which particular university. Tag clouds are also offered for individual scholars, thus helping to identify principal investigators in a specific field of research.[10]

Journals, citations, co-authors

In addition to the set of values mentioned above, Scholar Chart provides lists of the most popular journals that Finnish scholars are publishing in. The journals are organized at country, university and scholar levels. The work of each individual scholar is also illustrated with a graphical representation of absolute number of articles for the 36-month period. In addition, the most common co-authors of the scholar are listed and a direct link to Top Cited Articles citation search is provided. Also, article-level linking is used for Google Scholar and HubMed citations.

Scholar Chart is an innovative, constantly auto-updating alerting tool. It is an easy-to-use system for keeping count of Finnish medical articles published in the best international journals. Scholar Chart is an example of how libraries can add value with mashups and, in this case, promote the visibility of the research results produced by universities and their scholars.

Top Cited Articles

Top Cited Articles[11] lists in real time the most-cited articles from Finnish universities. Again, the lists can be chosen at university and national level. Browsing of different disciplines is also possible and the date range is the last 10 years. Author search is available and direct linking to search results is possible. The linking is also exploited in the Scholar Chart mashup. The citation information of the service comes from the Scopus[12] database (Elsevier B. V.) through the Scopus API.[13] An application programming interface (API)[14] is a source-code interface that an operating system or service provides to support requests made by computer programs. Access to an API should be a requirement when libraries are negotiating with database vendors. Top Cited Articles is a free service, but when visiting outside the Scopus subscribers' network some of the author and abstract information may be truncated and restricted.

Social bookmarking

During the Scholar Chart mashup processing, the University of Helsinki scholars' articles are also attached to the most important academic social bookmarking sites, i.e. CiteULike,[15] Connotea[16] and 2collab.[17] These sites are free services that help scholars to store and share references with their peers. By adding these bibliographical citations proactively, the Library is helping researchers to disseminate awareness of their research results to the growing global academic community who are working with the latest Web 2.0 technology.

Facebook

Some of the most important University of Helsinki articles are highlighted on Facebook.[18] They are hand picked during the mashup processing from the most prestigious journals, such as *Nature, Nature Genetics, Nature Medicine, New England Journal of Medicine, Lancet* and *BMJ*. In addition, much emphasis is put on the open access publications from PLoS (Public Library of Science) and BMC (BioMed Central).

MyTerkko

Another type of mashup are services that draw together content and tools from a wide range of services. MyTerkko[19] is an advanced Web 2.0 service for medical professionals. It consists of widgets that can be moved around the screen, extended and collapsed, and even removed if the widget is of no use to the customer. In addition to the traditional and most-used medical services that are assembled in MyTerkko, the user can gather further, supplementary Web 2.0 tools into the same interface – for example RSS feeds from FeedNavigator – or combine other feeds using Feed Builder application. The MyLinks widget opens up the possibility of adding and sharing users' own relevant links. Libraries should not limit their services to the interfaces that commercial database vendors are offering, but should integrate them into library applications in a genuine Web 2.0 way.

Future

Mashups, like the Scholar Chart, Top Cited Articles and MyTerkko services, offer new possibilities for libraries to innovate and create unequalled services. However, in addition to RSS feeds, more access to database APIs is needed. For example, the Scopus database is actively offering its application programming interface to be used with library mashups (13). Also, the Library needs to be proactive in relation to emerging technologies and try to promote new services within its own academic community or, in many cases, offer applications that are free to use for everyone.

Conclusions

The vision of the Scholar Chart service is to promote scholarly work published within the medical and health sciences discipline in Finland. It is freely available to users and is updated almost completely automatically. In addition, it offers highly interesting and at the same time somewhat controversial rankings of various measures, such as average Impact Factors and SCImago Journal Ranks. In conclusion, Scholar Chart, with its extension applications like Top Cited Articles, Facebook and social bookmarking, is helping Finnish medical scholars to make their contributions more visible and accessible to the global community of medical scholars.

References

1 Virtual Journal of Helsinki Medical Research [homepage on the internet], Helsinki: Terkko – National Library of Health Sciences, c2000–2005, www.terkko.helsinki.fi/vjhmr/.

2 Lund Medical Faculty Monthly, [homepage on the internet], Lund: Lund University, c2010, www.lmfm.med.lu.se/.

3 Wikipedia: RSS, [database on the internet], San Francisco (CA): Wikimedia Foundation Inc., c2010, http://en.wikipedia.org/wiki/RSS.

4 FeedNavigator, [database on the internet], Helsinki: Terkko – Meilahti Campus Library, c2010, www.terkko.helsinki.fi/feednavigator/.

5 PubMed, [database on the internet], Bethesda (MD): National Center for Biotechnology Information, c2010, www.ncbi.nlm.nih.gov/sites/entrez.

6 FeedNavigator: Helsinki University Scholar Channel, [database on the internet], Helsinki: Terkko – Meilahti Campus Library, c2010, www.terkko.helsinki.fi/feednavigator/?c=Tutkijat+/+Helsinki.

7 Scholar Chart, [database on the internet], Helsinki: Terkko – Meilahti Campus Library, c2010, www.terkko.helsinki.fi/scholarchart/.

8 Journal Citation Reports®, [homepage on the internet], Philadelphia (PA): The Thomson Corp., c2010, http://scientific.thomson.com/products/jcr/.

9 SJR – SCImago Journal and Country Rank, [homepage on the internet], Granada: SCImago Research Group, University of Granada, c2010, www.scimagojr.com.

10 OpenCalais [homepage on the internet], Philadelphia (PA): The Thomson Corp., c2010, www.opencalais.com/.

11 Top Cited Articles, [database on the internet], Helsinki: Terkko – Meilahti Campus Library, c2010, www.terkko.helsinki.fi/topcited/.

12 Scopus, [homepage on the internet], Amsterdam: Elsevier B. V., c2010, www.scopus.com/home.url.

13 Scopus API, [homepage on the internet], Amsterdam: Elsevier B. V., c2010, http://searchapi.scopus.com/.

14 Wikipedia: Application programming interface, [database on the internet], San Francisco (CA): Wikimedia Foundation Inc., c2010, http://en.wikipedia.org/wiki/Application_programming_interface.

15 CiteULike, [database on the internet], Bristol, UK, c2010, www.citeulike.org/.

16 Connotea, [database on the internet], London, UK: Nature Publishing Group, c2010, www.connotea.org/.

17 2collab, [database on the internet], Amsterdam: Elsevier B. V., c2010, www.2collab.com/.

18 Terkko@Facebook, [homepage on the internet], Helsinki: Terkko – Meilahti Campus Library, c2010, www.facebook.com/terkko.

19 MyTerkko, [homepage on the internet], Helsinki: Terkko – Meilahti Campus Library, c2010, www.terkko.helsinki.fi/.

CHAPTER 12

Twitter in a hospital library

Hannah Prince

Introduction

As the manager of a hospital library, I started exploring Twitter as a way of communicating with my library users and potential users. Many libraries are using Twitter in lots of different ways; this chapter describes my experience and some of the decisions I have made.

My library

The library I work in is based in the Princess Alexandra Hospital, a small general hospital in Harlow, just outside London. We support staff and students in all the NHS organizations in Harlow and its surrounding small towns and villages: the hospital itself, local mental health units, clinics and GP surgeries. In total, we have around 5000 potential users but the majority do not make regular use of the library.

Our wide geographical area and the increasing time pressures on NHS staff both contribute to an increased interest in providing library services electronically. However, the demographic and the spread of technology usage in the community are as wide as they could be: from medical students to managers, nurses to porters, and from those with the latest smartphone to those whose children help them search the web.

Starting to use Twitter

Setting up a Twitter account is technically very straightforward: you can create an account in a few minutes by registering a unique username at www.twitter.com. There are excellent guides available online to setting up your account (see the section on Further reading).

When I started using Twitter for the library, there were a few points I considered:

- whether it was the right approach for what I wanted to achieve
- who the target audience should be
- what sort of information to share

- what other uses could be made of the format
- whether my employer would be comfortable with my use of this informal way of communicating.

In the light of experience, I would recommend that librarians who start to use Twitter should also consider:

- how best to access Twitter to suit your work pattern
- on what terms to engage with other people on Twitter
- how to resolve questions about what you should and shouldn't 'tweet' (post to Twitter)
- how to publicize a Twitter account among your target audience
- how to evaluate the impact of your work on Twitter.

Why use Twitter?

Contrarily, I first looked into Twitter because I wanted a blog.

I wanted a blog because I wanted some way of getting information to library users about interesting new resources, events or ideas. Frustratingly, I found that I could not find time to regularly compose a few paragraphs. Twitter appealed because I could quickly pass information on, commenting when I wanted to but with no obligation to think of something extra to say. Every post is limited to 140 characters, which is just long enough for a thought and perhaps a link.

Twitter's simplicity is one of its key features. Once an account has been created and a few basics have been understood, it is possible to use it productively without ever investigating further. 'Following' another Twitter account makes everything that person 'tweets' (writes) appear on your Twitter homepage (your 'timeline') for you to read. When you tweet something yourself, it is readable by everyone who follows you, and by anyone in the world who searches Twitter for a word you have used. It is common to pass on another person's tweet by 'retweeting' it: posting it yourself, acknowledging the original source.

My feed is aimed at my library users, not at other librarians or providers of information. I decided early on that I would pick a target audience and stick to it. Many other librarians successfully combine spreading information and interacting with others: Twitter is an ideal place to join a community of people sharing ideas, reply to others' tweets, ask and answer questions.

I was not expecting that a large number of my audience used Twitter directly. I was interested in engaging with those who did, but primarily wanted an easy way to update a 'news from the library' feed that I could use on the Trust intranet.

As I started using Twitter, I discovered some further uses; they include:

- Keeping up to date myself: oddly, this had not occurred to me when I started, but as more UK health organizations use Twitter, it is a very effective way to keep up.

- Getting information from live events I cannot attend: increasingly, people are tweeting from conferences and workshops, which gives a flavour of the discussions. A book on this topic for presenters was published recently (Atkinson, 2010).
- Raising awareness of library services by doing something unexpected: there is still surprise value in having a librarian talk about Twitter, which can help to make potential library users realize that their library provides more services than the immediately obvious.

Making it useful

Some people tweet every few minutes, some every few months. The frequency with which someone tweets is sometimes a way that others decide whether or not to follow them. Tweeting too much can be more off-putting than tweeting too little. This is because each tweet appears in followers' timelines in chronological order, so it is more noticeable that someone is constantly tweeting than that they have not posted for a while.

As I intended my Twitter feed to double as a news feed from the library, I decided that I needed to aim to tweet at least once a day. In practice, this means that some days I post a few things and other days not at all.

When using Twitter, it is worth bearing in mind that you are not your followers' only source of information. Twitter is designed to pull together lots of sources into one place, so there is no need to attempt to cover everything. Some things I wanted to cover regularly were casualties of time: I decided that it was better to accept this and keep passing on useful things when I could, rather than to give up because I could not be comprehensive.

One thing I am sure about is the need to add value. Ways to be useful to my followers include:

- acting as a filter on other accounts: retweeting one or two interesting things from the accounts I follow, like an article about an area I know my hospital is developing
- commenting on the things I read: saying who I think might find a link particularly useful, or adding my reflection on the issues raised
- talking about what I am doing and thinking about, to give insight into the work the library does.

It would be easy to get into the habit of just doing the first of these; I think it is important to try to do all three.

Adding commentary generally means giving some personal opinion. My name appears in the account biography, but tweets from this account are from the library, not from me personally. I try to pitch the tone as though I were talking directly to a library user: professional but friendly. This tone seems to suit the format.

Some of the things I have tweeted about include:

- Contents of the newest issue of the Lancet, BMJ or other major journals.
- An interesting journal article or website I have just found.
- A new White Paper or report.
- Announcing the publication of the latest Cochrane Library update.
- Passing on someone else's comment on a UK healthcare issue.
- A new tool or workaround for searching online.
- A link to a list of useful websites I have just put together, sometimes directly after the topic has been covered in a local meeting.
- Library closure days.
- A new Annual Evidence Update from one of the NHS Evidence Specialist Collections.
- New books in the library.
- Events in the hospital, or national or regional events.
- News from the hospital. This might include a link to newly published ratings, or other pieces of interest to staff. The hospital's communications department has its own Twitter account for news for the public.
- On National Poetry Day, a link to a health-related poet.
- A note that an e-journal website is down. Many companies monitor Twitter for mentions of their product, so it can be an additional way of alerting them to a problem.

Ethical issues

I have been surprised by the way that using Twitter has made me think about ethics; it was not something I had anticipated when I started experimenting with a web tool. It seems obvious now: censorship happens when choices are made to exclude something, and a 140-character format forces the omission of a lot of detail.

Some choices are related to my decision to tweet as @pahlibrary rather than under my own name. This can make mentioning 'in the news' topics difficult; healthcare is an area where news, politics and ethics often collide. There have been comments I have not posted and links I have not passed on when I have not felt able to be neutral, but I do not want to be seen as placing my employer on one side of a debate.

It is also hard to summarize an idea in a short space without losing meaning. I have grown more careful of commenting on newly published research, as I realize how easy it is to dramatically misrepresent something by leaving out relevant information.

Productivity and access at work

I am able to access Twitter at work. Some workplace IT policies block access, perhaps on the assumption that it is used primarily for socializing.

I do feel strongly that gathering information and pushing it to where it is needed is a fundamental part of my job. I had talked to my hospital's Head of Communications before I set up my feed, so I was confident that tweeting from the library would not be rejected in principle. However, I started using Twitter quietly, as an unpublicized experiment, so that by the time any sceptics in my organization saw it, it would have developed some value.

Twitter can be a great thief of time. If you follow more than a few people, just reading recent tweets takes time. Following links will take longer, so it is important to consider how to balance it with the rest of your workload. To stay completely up to date, I would have to leave Twitter open on my desktop all day. Personally, I cannot do this and concentrate on anything else. Instead, I accept that I will not be able to read everything and allot just a short period in the day to check in, skim recent tweets and post something myself. Mobile access makes it easier to catch up at home, when I am so inclined.

There are a few useful tools that make it quicker to post something on Twitter. Links to URL shorteners and a 'Share on Twitter' browser button can save a few minutes and make it much easier to share something interesting. There are a number of alternative interfaces for Twitter, available as web services or for download to your computer, which add functionality; some allow you to filter incoming tweets or sort the people you follow into lists, both useful tools if you follow a large number of people.

The original Twitter website is not designed for use with Internet Explorer version 6. This browser is the only one I can use at work, a common situation in NHS organizations at the time of writing. Functionality is not currently affected beyond some non-ideal location of pictures on the screen, but it may be that developments to the interface will make it harder to use with the old browser. If so, alternative interfaces may become more necessary.

API, applications and automation

It is arguable that one of the reasons for Twitter's popular success is its open application programming interface (API). This allows developers to use its code to make web and mobile applications (apps) that link in with Twitter. Many services have taken advantage of this, resulting in a huge variety of extra ways to use Twitter: there are more than 50,000 registered Twitter apps, and websites exist just to index them.

Some apps offer more efficient ways of using Twitter itself: recommending followers, sending tweets to a specified group, or presenting tweets as a newspaper or digest. Others link your Twitter account to external services: many people link their account with their Facebook account or blog, so updating one updates the other. It is possible to link Twitter to your Google calendar, your e-mail, your browser and your Delicious account. In a training workshop full of people with mobile phones, you could ask everyone to tweet their answer to a question with a hashtag (a way of marking up a keyword in a tweet, by preceding it with a #) and use an app called Twitterfall to display the answers on the screen. There are apps to track packages, send yourself reminders or share files. Apps develop and die off regularly; it is best to accept this, be alert and be ready to move on.

One type of app allows you to schedule a tweet to be posted to Twitter at a time and date of your choosing. I am currently using an app of this type called Socialoomph. Scheduling or automating tweets requires some caution to avoid their looking like spam: it is worth reading Twitter's regulations and thinking about what would annoy you in someone you were following. Some people like to use scheduling to spread tweets out through the day and avoid overloading their followers, others to make sure that an event or release is tweeted on the day it happens. I am planning a publicity campaign on recent book purchases that tweets one book a day, using a URL shortener for the link to the library catalogue and a hashtag to make it easy to find just those tweets. Then I can create an RSS feed for the hashtag and display the feed on a library web page.

Twitter language and etiquette

Any social media site has its own etiquette and language and you will always find blog posts describing a correct way to behave. Twitter has lent itself to a language that can sound rather saccharine, but has the benefit that there is no obligation to use it: you do not have to say 'tweeple' if it makes you feel silly.

Twitter is uncomplicated, but there are some basic things to get right. For example, retweeting – passing on someone else's tweet to your own followers, with or without a comment – is a fundamental way of using Twitter. As you are using someone else's idea, it is polite to attribute it; fortunately, this is simple to do by using the Retweet function or by adding 'RT' and the Twitter username of the original tweeter. Adding 'via' or 'HT' (heard through) to a username is a way of acknowledging a source you are not directly quoting.

People including links in a tweet will often use a URL shortener like bit.ly. If you have found a website through someone else's link, it is nice to use the same shortened URL: some shorteners provide hit counts, which is a way for the original poster to evaluate their reach.

Two-way communication

Two-way communication is one of the things Twitter does well, but in a singular way: direct messaging allows individual messages between people who follow each other, but most conversations are public. To get a particular person's attention, you use their

Twitter username in a tweet (called an @mention or @reply, because you put @ in front of the username).

I found myself using Twitter as a one-way service: posting tweets, hoping others would read them, but not engaging with other people beyond retweeting them. This was a side effect of using it as a newsfeed into our intranet page: I did not want a casual reader of the intranet page to find a reply that made no sense out of context. It also fits the model of checking in once a day rather than being always online.

It is occasionally frustrating not to join in completely, and does mean missing out on some of the benefits of Twitter. One solution is to respond to others in a way that makes sense to people reading; another is to retweet the original comment, then reply. I have not yet experimented with inviting library users to use @mentions to send questions; offering it as an official 'ask the librarian' type service would mean having to be more careful about checking the account regularly.

There is always the solution of setting up a separate, personal account. I did this during the 2010 UK general election, which was a huge event on Twitter: it was possible to 'watch' the debates and election night on Twitter as much as on television.

Getting information from Twitter

Twitter is a place to find information as well as disseminate it. As well as receiving information from the tweets of people you follow, you can search Twitter using its own search tool or a number of third-party search engines. Many Twitter search tools will allow you to save a search or set up an RSS feed from a search. I use an RSS feed to keep up with mentions of my hospital on Twitter.

Publicizing a Twitter feed

I have more followers from outside my local area than from within. This is partly because my Twitter account is on a list of UK librarians put together by Phil Bradley at tweepml.com, and people often use the 'follow everyone on this list' function. This is an excellent way to get noticed: Twitter puts value on personal recommendation, so being on the list of a popular tweeter is useful, as is being retweeted or namechecked by other users. Follow Friday or FF is a Twitter institution where people tweet the usernames of others they recommend (generally on a Friday, hence the name).

Proactive ways of bringing yourself to other people's attention on Twitter include following people (they will get an e-mail with a link to your account, and can choose to follow you back), retweeting people (they will see that you have retweeted them) or simply searching for other people who mention topics of interest or are based in your area.

There are also the standard methods of publicity: including a link to your Twitter feed in an e-mail signature and library leaflets or mentioning it in internal newsletters and talks. The more it fits alongside your other publicity or current awareness activities, the higher its profile will be in your organization.

Conclusion: evaluating Twitter's usefulness

Whether using Twitter is actually worth the time invested has to be an individual calculation for each user.

For myself, there are positives and negatives. I am still finding that the majority of my followers are not my target audience. I think the low-key way I started using Twitter has persisted for too long and I need to publicize the feed and investigate more uses to make it more worth the time invested. Although Twitter's use is still expanding and becoming more mainstream, it could continue to be the case that individual clinicians do not use it. In that case, we may see the maximum benefits only if I use Twitter to gather information and then use the linked web services to push the feed to library users through alternative means.

On the positive side, I am already glad to have the newsfeed to our intranet page; I am looking forward to experimenting with additional ways to use and publicize the library feed, and by following a range of interesting people I am gathering far more information about healthcare, librarianship and medical education than I used to. I am getting a small publicity bump when I mention it, I feel like I am part of a network of people interested in the things I am interested in, and the time investment has really been very small.

There are ways to measure impact more precisely: you can track click-throughs from links you post, count local followers and retweets, or use an app which collects Twitter metrics.

Ultimately, I would encourage anyone interested in health information to experiment with Twitter: for a tool so simple, it is surprisingly powerful.

Further reading
Print material

Atkinson, C. (2010) *The Backchannel: how audiences are using Twitter and social media and changing presentations forever*, New Riders.

Bradley, P. (2009) Gathering Followers Twitter in the Skies . . ., *Library & Information Update*, (April), 34–7.

Defebbo, D. M., Mihlrad, L. and Strong, M. A. (2009) Microblogging for Medical Libraries and Librarians, *Journal of Electronic Resources in Medical Libraries*, **6**(3), 211–23.

Giustini, D. and Wright, M. (2009) Twitter: an introduction to microblogging for health librarians, *Journal of the Canadian Health Libraries Association* (*JCHLA*), **30** (1), 11–17, http://article.pubs.nrc-cnrc.gc.ca/RPAS/RPViewDoc?_handler_= HandleInitialGet&calyLang=eng&journal=jchla&volume=30&articleFile= c09-009.pdf.

Milstein, S. (2009) Twitter for Libraries (and Librarians), *Computers in Libraries*, **29**(5), 17–18, www.infotoday.com/cilmag/may09/Milstein.shtml.

van Zyl, A. S. (2009) The Impact of Social Networking 2.0 on Organizations, *The Electronic Library*, **27** (6), 906–18.

Online

Phil Bradley has an excellent blogpost introducing some ideas for using Twitter in libraries: http://philbradley.typepad.com/phil_bradleys_weblog/2009/01/using-twitter-in-libraries.html. It is worth searching this blog for other information on Twitter, as the author has written on the subject several times and is always interesting; see also the article below.

Twitter itself provides a guide for businesses: http://business.twitter.com/twitter101. Many of these points are relevant for libraries and information providers.

Museum Buddies, an MLA-related project, has some brief advice on using Twitter as a publicity tool: www.mubu.org.uk/support/category/twitter.

Services mentioned in this chapter

bit.ly, http://bit.ly

SocialOomph, www.socialoomph.com

TweepML.com, http://tweepml.org

Twitterfall, www.twitterfall.com

One index of Twitter apps is Twitdom: http://twitdom.com.

There are a number of apps that will give you Twitter metrics: one to try is www.twitteranalyzer.com, or see http://twitdom.com/tag/statistics/.

CHAPTER 13

Using Web 2.0 to facilitate staff development

Andrew Booth, Anthea Sutton and Andy Tattersall

Introduction

Recent years have seen an increasing imperative for health librarians and information professionals to demonstrate that they possess, and use, mechanisms for 'keeping current' (Health Executive Advisory Group, 2004; Cunningham, 2010). As the speed of organizational and technical change becomes increasingly rapid, the requisite skill base covers an ever wider range of competencies (captured in the acronym COMPLIANT). Increasing user expectations, coupled with demands for quality, accountability and efficacy of practice, further emphasize the need to demonstrate strategies for periodic refreshment of skills and knowledge (Lacey and Booth, 2003). At the same time, conferences and workshops, traditional routes for acquiring such updates, are becoming less accessible as budgetary constraints and lack of time, combined with the need to provide continuity of front-line service, limit opportunities for staff to attend external training courses. E-learning, delivered via the web and facilitated by an increasing array of Web 2.0 technologies, offers the prospect of delivering staff development to library staff in the workplace (Ayiku et al., 2005).

Requirements for staff development

Our review of workplace-based e-learning identified five major themes: (1) peer communication, (2) flexibility, (3) support, (4) knowledge validation and (5) course presentation and design (Booth et al., 2009). The implications of these themes are as follows:

1 E-learners working in isolation typically need to be able to interact with other learners and to receive social support for learning.
2 Pressures of work make it more difficult to establish a routine for learning; deadlines for interaction or for assessment must be as flexible as possible.
3 Workplace-based e-learners lack the reassurance that is provided by face-to-face interaction with teaching staff and require speedy and efficient support in response to questions.

4 Mechanisms for checking knowledge are essential if e-learners are to verify their own learning and understanding *throughout* the learning module, not just at the end of the module.

5 Course materials must be well presented and easy to navigate, particularly as workplace learners typically learn opportunistically, in bite-sized chunks, rather than enjoying the luxury of protected study time.

How Web 2.0 measures up

It is immediately apparent that Web 2.0 technology has much to offer in meeting the five identified needs of workplace-based learners rehearsed above. The interactivity and ease of use of blog and wiki technologies facilitate communication with (Grassley and Bartoletti, 2009) and peer support from fellow learners (Moen et al., 2009). Placing resources on the web means that, in addition to receiving regular course e-mails, learners have an immediate way of reviewing past content and catching up, using recent materials that hang off the framework of a course curriculum. A central resource for each course can be supplemented with supporting materials that stand in for tutor support at times when the course team is unavailable. Quizzes, formative feedback (as the course goes along) and an acceptable turn-around time for student enquiries reduces the weight placed on end-of-module feedback. Finally, the 'What You See Is What You Get' (WYSIWYG) nature of many blog and wiki technologies makes it correspondingly easier to produce attractively presented resources that are more intuitive to navigate.

The use of Web 2.0 for staff development not only includes library-specific initiatives but is also informed by wider developments in health, medical and nursing education (Kamel Boulos, Maramba and Wheeler, 2006; Kamel Boulos and Wheeler, 2007; Lemley and Burnham, 2009) as well as in education more broadly (Weller et al., 2005). More evaluation and sharing of experience are needed in order to build the evidence base for the usefulness of these tools within the context of staff development. Much collective learning is currently being achieved through small-scale case studies, such as the one presented below.

Case study: FOLIO/FOLIOz Programme

A team at ScHARR Information Resources designs, develops and delivers a programme of work-based e-learning courses for library and information professionals in the UK (in collaboration with the Strategic Health Authority Library Leads (SHALL)) and in Australia and New Zealand (in collaboration with the Australian Library and Information Association (ALIA)). This programme is called FOLIO – Facilitated Online Learning as an Interactive Opportunity – with FOLIOz being the southern hemisphere variant.

A fundamental low-technology philosophy means that the eight-week courses are delivered primarily by e-mail. However, this minimalist approach has provided good opportunities for an incremental approach to the introduction of supporting web materials – such as wiki pages, discussion forums, podcasts, online quizzes, along with other uses of Web 2.0 technologies. The focus on ease of access, using online tools that are freely available, and ease of use, with the emphasis being on the learning dynamic rather than on technical proficiency, has kept the FOLIO courses true to their originating principles.

Peer communication, and indeed collaboration, is an important element of each course, with participants encouraged to interact in buddy groups. This contributes to an effective and enjoyable learning experience. What we had not appreciated, however, was demand from participants themselves to be able to interact more generally, and not simply for task-related purposes. In response to this demand we have built up a resource base of materials to support participant-initiated interactions to complement 'official' course communications. This ten-part resource is housed on the University of Sheffield's own collaborative space, uSpace (http://uspace.shef.ac.uk/clearspace/groups/folio-group), and covers many of the most useful Web 2.0 tools to enable learners to communicate and collaborate efficiently. Topics include:

1 Useful study resources and tools – introduction to Web 2.0
2 Going beyond Google for searching
3 Bookmark your resources anywhere
4 Create feeds from useful resources
5 Manage your references online
6 Create your own web pages
7 Chat with your fellow students using discussion forums and instant messaging
8 Send, save and share files without using large e-mail attachments
9 Write your own Blog/Diary
10 Useful websites and tools.

In addition, supplementary materials include 'Useful video tutorials', comprising instructional resources derived primarily from YouTube.

In addition to this online, in-house uSpace tool, which facilitates the creation of online documents, hosting of files, discussions and blogging, the FOLIO team continues to use external wiki tools such as PBWorks. Materials from FOLIO courses are thus available not only to course participants but also for use by any other interested parties. This ease of access, without requiring the mediation of a facilitator, is particularly important for Australian and New Zealand participants, for whom there is a significant, but nevertheless tolerable, 'time gap' between the despatch of instructions (between 4 p.m. and 5 p.m. UK time) and the support team's being back in the office at 9 a.m. (UK) the following day.

Why use Web 2.0?

By employing online tools and harnessing Web 2.0 technologies, course providers can effectively support international, workplace-based learners. Benefits include:

- Helping learners to communicate effectively with peers across geographical and time zone boundaries.
- Encouraging learners to use Web 2.0 tools in their professional careers, and thus to become a resource to their organization and colleagues.
- Allowing learners to build up their own personal learning networks and thus to share ideas and concepts away from the 'official' educational environment.
- Employing social software to stimulate reflective practice (Hall and Davison, 2007) and to capture and store knowledge in a way that is easily transferable.

In reality, our courses, and indeed those of others, cannot be described as *purely* Web 2.0 courses. What we are able to do is integrate existing resources, such as JISCMail discussion lists, with their own increasing functionality, with Web 2.0 tools so as to provide a low-cost alternative to off-the-shelf virtual learning environments. In a sense, Web 2.0 provides the 'glue' with which the various components are fused together into an almost seamless course package (Kamel Boulos and Wheeler, 2007).

Lessons learned

Use of Web 2.0 technologies has not been without its difficulties and challenges. Most courses open to a trickle of e-mails alerting us that some participants wrongly believe that they must log in to the wiki simply to access materials, as opposed to authoring them. Similarly, within the pressured environment of workplace-based learning, the distinction between a facilitator-controlled wiki hosting (and protecting the integrity of) the course materials and a participant-owned wiki where participants do log in and post arguments either in favour of or against a topic for debate occasionally becomes a nicety that passes some by. For this reason it is essential to ensure that learners are aware of the tools available to them and of the pros and cons of using each tool; and for them to be reassured that instruction and help are available online. We have found it helpful to outline a learning protocol at the beginning of the course so as to create realistic expectations regarding the interactions required and an awareness of appropriate and inappropriate patterns of communication.

A knowledge of participants *and* technologies has been essential, so that we can be as sure as we can that the tools we use – and ask participants to use – are actually capable of delivering the outputs we want. Such knowledge has been acquired over several years as we analyse extensive data from the mandatory feedback forms received for each course.

Finally, we have discovered the value of making the online resources do much of the hard work for us. To a large extent, the value of FOLIO courses is not so much in the creation of new learning resources – although we naturally take pride in our imaginative and realistic scenarios for exploiting shared learning – but in harnessing many existing resources in an appropriate and productive way. To provide just one example, embedding a YouTube video (such as a scene from *The Office* on staff appraisal) into e-learning support resources offers not only time savings for the course tutor but also ease of use for the student. Such videos can subsequently be shared as reusable objects through embedding and social bookmarking. Again, the focus is not on gratuitous entertainment but on stimulating tightly directed learning points as a starting point for professional reflection.

If we had known then . . .

The body of knowledge and good practice around the use of Web 2.0 technologies for staff development is continually expanding. Stimulated by accounts from others using blog technologies to share learning from conferences (Goodfellow and Graham, 2007), we can reflect on whether requiring each participant to keep a blog, as an alternative to the current Word portfolio submission, may be a more appropriate output from each FOLIO course. Indeed, such an approach could help participants to follow up course participation by applying learning to their practice, and sharing lessons learned with their colleagues. Similarly, we are monitoring with interest attempts to use Twitter for formative evaluation (Stieger and Burger, 2010).

FOLIO staff members have developed creative solutions in response to pressing and immediate practical problems. This has the advantage of keeping learning as the focus, rather than being distracted by the enabling technology (Booth, 2007). However, it also means that many solutions are constrained by the limitations of our own knowledge and therefore represent 'making do' rather than necessarily being the 'best of all possible solutions' (Sandars, 2006). Frequently, too, we have to make compromises between what is optimal and what is easily achievable. For example, while it is technically feasible to embed a slide-specific segment of commentary into each PowerPoint slide in an online presentation, this is necessarily time consuming. Providing a single podcast commentary, including the spoken instructions 'Advance to next slide', may be less elegant and user friendly for participants, but is more commensurate with the resources available to our courses.

Conclusion

Intrinsically, Web 2.0 technologies can be seen to adhere to adult learning principles such as enquiry-based learning, group learning, experiential learning and interaction (Brixey and Warren, 2009; Gross and Leslie, 2008). They facilitate a role for the instructor as a 'guide from the side'. As such, we might contrast this with early-generation web technologies whereby the Web 1.0 model of the static page corresponded closely to a 'sage on the stage' approach to instruction. In this sense, technology and pedagogy can be seen as evolving synergistically.

Furthermore, Web 2.0 technologies have the unique properties of being both the means for delivering staff development on any topic and a topic for staff development in their own right (Rethlefsen et al., 2009). As we deliver the FOLIO course on 'Introduction to e-learning', for example, we can be secure in the knowledge that participants are learning by doing as well as learning by reading. Indeed, participants in any FOLIO course are equipping themselves with useful skills and experience in using the available technologies. In addition, they are learning to cultivate empathy for those users who are themselves undergoing workplace-based e-learning and having to manage the delicate balance in the conflict between work and learning!

References

Ayiku, L., Sutton, A., Turner, A., Booth, A. and O'Rourke, A. (2005) Meeting the CPD Needs of the E-Librarian. In Genoni, P. and Walton, G. (eds), *Continuing Professional Development – Preparing for New Roles in Libraries: a voyage of discovery*, Sixth World Conference on Continuing Professional Development and Workplace Learning for the Library and Information Professions, Walter de Gruyter/K. G. Saur, 126–36.

Booth, A. (2007) Blogs, Wikis and Podcasts: the 'evaluation bypass' in action? *Health Information and Libraries Journal*, **24** (4), 298–302.

Booth, A., Carroll, C., Papaioannou, D., Sutton, A. and Wong, R. (2009) Applying Findings from a Systematic Review of Workplace-based E-learning: implications for health information professionals, *Health Information and Libraries Journal*, **26** (1), 4–21.

Brixey, J. J. and Warren, J. J. (2009) Creating Experiential Learning Activities Using Web 2.0 tools and technologies: a case study, *Studies in Health Technology and Informatics*, **146**, 613–17.

Cunningham, K. (2010) The Hidden Costs of Keeping Current: technology and libraries, *Journal of Library Administration*, **50** (3), 217–35.

Goodfellow, T. and Graham, S. (2007) The Blog as a High-impact Institutional Communication Tool, *The Electronic Library*, **25** (4), 395–400.

Grassley, J. S. and Bartoletti, R. (2009) Wikis and Blogs: tools for online interaction, *Nurse Educator*, **34** (5), 209–13.

Gross, J. and Leslie, L. (2008) Twenty-three Steps to Learning Web 2.0 Technologies in an Academic Library, *The Electronic Library*, **26** (6), 790–802.

Hall, H. and Davison, B. (2007) Social Software as Support in Hybrid Learning Environments: the value of the blog as a tool for reflective learning and peer support, *Library and Information Science Research*, **29**, 163–87.

Health Executive Advisory Group (2004) *Future Proofing the Profession: the report of the Health Executive Advisory Group*, CILIP.

Kamel Boulos, M. N. and Wheeler, S. (2007) The Emerging Web 2.0 Social Software: an enabling suite of sociable technologies in health and health care education, *Health Information and Libraries Journal*, **24** (1), 2–23.

Kamel Boulos, M. N., Maramba, I. and Wheeler, S. (2006) Wikis, Blogs and Podcasts: a new generation of web-based tools for virtual collaborative clinical practice and education, *BMC Medical Education*, **6**, 41, http://www.ncbi.nlm.nih.gov/pmc/articles/PMC1564136/pdf/1472-6920-6-41.pdf.

Lacey, T. and Booth, A. (2003) *Education, Training and Development for NHS Librarians: Supporting E-learning: a review commissioned by the National electronic Library for Health Librarian Development Programme*, University of Sheffield, ScHARR (School of Health and Related Research).

Lemley, T. and Burnham, J. F. (2009) Web 2.0 Tools in Medical and Nursing School Curricula, *Journal of the Medical Library Association*, **97** (1), 50–2.

Moen, A., Smørdal, O. and Sem, I. (2009) Web-based Resources for Peer Support – Opportunities and Challenges, *Studies in Health Technology and Informatics*, **150**, 302–6.

Rethlefsen, M. L., Piorun, M. and Prince, J. D. (2009) Teaching Web 2.0 Technologies using Web 2.0 Technologies, *Journal of the Medical Library Association*, **97**(4), 253–9.

Sandars, J. (2006) Twelve Tips for Using Blogs and Wikis in Medical Education, *Medical Teacher*, **28** (8), 680–2.

Stieger, S. and Burger, C. (2010) Let's Go Formative: continuous student ratings with Web 2.0 application Twitter, *Cyberpsychology and Behavior: the impact of the internet, multimedia and virtual reality on behavior and society*, **13** (2), 163–7.

Weller, M., Pegler, C. and Mason, R. (2005) Use of Innovative Technologies on an Elearning Course, *Internet and Higher Education*, **8**, 61–71.

PART 4

The future

CHAPTER 14

Web 3.0 and health librarians: what does the future hold?

Allan Cho and Dean Giustini

Introduction

In a 2001 *Scientific American* article, Sir Tim Berners-Lee shares his vision for the world wide web which he believes will solve most of humankind's 'most complex problems' (Berners-Lee et al., 2001). In this chapter, we provide an update on the evolution of Web 3.0 and Berners-Lee's ideas for a Semantic Web – two separate terms that many believe are synonymous, while others dispute if they even exist. In addition, we reflect on what Web 3.0 means for health librarians and whether there are new roles for us in shaping its future.

Web 3.0 is more than semantics

A word of warning: both the Semantic Web and Web 3.0 lack clear definitions (see Glossary), yet these terms are widely and interchangeably used. For us, Web 3.0 refers to the third decade of the web and the Semantic Web is simply part of that; however, this interpretation is also disputed (Anderson and Rainie, 2010). The experts cannot agree on a name, a definition or whether Web 3.0 exists. What is important for librarians to remember is that Web 3.0 is not a whole new internet space but a group of trends that extends the web's functionality by:

- translating the web into a language that can be read and categorized by computers
- applying the technologies of the Semantic Web to improve how information is found
- creating a way to link to documents ('to create linked data') through artificial intelligence (AI) and machine-based reasoning
- integrating three-dimensional (3D), virtual and physical worlds into an immersive web experience.

Consider for a moment that the current web is evolving from Web 2.0 into a mobile and immersive medium (Lippincott, 2010). Part of the (r)evolution includes geolocation tools like Foursquare and virtual worlds like Second Life. But conceptually, the next-generation web or 'web of data' as articulated by Berners-Lee and others looks back to an earlier model of documentation by Paul Otlet in the early 20th century (Wright, 2009) and to bibliographic control by Melvil Dewey and Antonio Panizzi in the 19th century (Carpenter, 2002). For the cutting edge in organizing and linking important information, what's old seems new again.

The Semantic Web in progress

> ... semantics comes from the Greek to give signs, meaning, or to make significant. Semantics refers to aspects of meaning as expressed in language or systems of signs. (Giustini, 2007)

In 2011, the Semantic Web is clearly a work in progress. A 2010 Pew Internet and American Life Project survey 'The fate of the Semantic Web' reported that 47% of 895 of the world's technology experts agreed with the statement 'by 2020, the semantic web envisioned by Tim Berners-Lee will not be as effective as its creators had hoped and average users will not have noticed much of a difference' (Anderson and Rainie, 2010). Conversely, the other experts seem to imply that in 2011 we are in a pre-semantic period, midway between Web 2.0 and Web 3.0 (Table 14.1).

Table 14.1 *The Semantic Web in progress*

Web 2.0	Web 3.0
'The social web'	'The Semantic Web'
Abundance of information	Abundance of meaning
Social media	Intelligent agents
The second decade, 2000–10	The third decade, 2010–20
Google as catalyst	Linked data as catalyst
Searching	Finding
Wisdom of crowds	Wisdom of semantic tools
Google's PageRank	Semantic search engines
HTML, SGML	HTML5, XML
Lawless, keywords, anarchic	Standards, metadata, protocols
Print and digital access	Born or *made* digital, open access (OA)

In reality, a few semantic search tools have already been released that provide a glimpse into the future (see Glossary). While some of these search tools remain in *beta*, they do show how semantic technologies can work when good data (and structure) are available to them in the languages of the World Wide Web Consortium (W3C) (Fazzinga and Lukasiewicz, 2010). For example, a semantic search engine will not work on web pages written in natural markup (Guha et al., 2003). Extensible markup languages such as XML (to format web pages) and standards developed by W3C are needed to create Semantic Web functionality (Marshall and Shipman, 2003). Although we do not yet have the supportive structure underneath, the deeper, more structured approach to information gathering that the Semantic Web represents stands in contrast, at least theoretically, to the superficial structure of the web as it exists today and the keyword search capabilities of our most popular search engines, Google, Yahoo! and Bing.

Ambient access to information

[In Web 3.0] search engines understand who you are, what you've been doing ... and where you'd like to go next. (Strickland, 2007)

In 2011, web technology is everywhere. Its pervasiveness is seen at universities, especially in the learning commons of most academic libraries, in business and government, and also when simply walking down a busy urban street where people are using their mobile devices. Smartphones provide new affordances such as ambient access to information, cloud computing or storage 'out there' on the web, not to mention other opportunities (Lippincott, 2010). For medical professionals, platforms such as Apple's iPhone and iPad, Blackberrys and Google's Android offer on-the-go convenience and communication in and out of the clinic. Wireless devices with high-speed access, high-resolution cameras and global positioning devices make it possible for health professionals to obtain information on demand, whenever it is needed.

Data are literally all around us. New social tools and phone applications afford a pervasive here-I-am visibility – information used by others to generalize our consumer habits and market products to us. Today, all kinds of inferences are made about our online habits from the activities we engage in online. Now that we are freed from our desktops, due to mobiles, simple tools such as Google Docs and wikis make it easy to create knowledge 'in the cloud'. A popular trend in social media is monitoring other people in the expectation that we will update our digital presence for others as much as possible. Locative tools such as Foursquare and Gowalla, inspired by Twitter, allow users to say where they are going, while sharing tips and inside information along the way. Together, these trends create the ubiquitous computing promised by Web 3.0.

Some cities in the USA are working towards being completely wireless. Wireless capability substantially increases how much we use mobiles, including plugging back into our physical world. Where static physical objects in the past had no special communicative or social affordances, when connected to computers in 'intelligent' ways, they become part of the 'Internet of things' (Atzori, Iera and Morabito, 2010). In the home, household appliances offer new potential by linking to mobile devices and a small computer, say in your fridge, to know when you need milk. The idea of machines being an extension of man's senses goes back to Marshall McLuhan in the 1960s, but the urge to connect all objects and devices looks forward to Web 3.0.

Some internet experts believe that connecting devices to physical objects requires innovative and expensive hardware (Silva, Mahfujur Rahman et al., 2008); others believe that connectivity can be realized through radio-frequency identification (RFID), quick-response (QR) codes and augmented-reality technology (Walsh, 2010). In this environment of hyper-reality, objects like books leave 'information shadows', evidence of their existence that is present in internet environments such as Amazon, eBay, or Twitter (O'Reilly and Battelle, 2009). Smart tools can now communicate with physical objects and reveal information beyond our perception:

> . . . you are walking down a street in Rome. Using the information from Google Maps, the system can give you recommendations for lunch or breakfast, depending on the time of the day and your personal preferences for food and beverages. You could have marks imposed on the street image to guide you to the Coliseum and then to a Chinese restaurant, and the phone number of the restaurant in case you want to make a reservation for two persons. And while visiting the Coliseum, information about the site is pulled from Wikipedia. (Corlain, 2009)

The above story illustrates how information technologies can be integrated to broaden our experience of the world. In Berners-Lee's article from 2001, a similar anecdote is used: using her hand-held device, Lucy asks her Semantic Web agent to provide information about her mother's prescription and how best to fill it. Using voice-enabled technology, she asks for a list of pharmacies within a 20-mile radius, including those with the best consumer rating scores, which she uses to place an order. Although this is a hypothetical situation, it illustrates what smart agents promise to do for us on the next-generation web.

Deep layers of meaning

> For hundreds of years, metadata was kept in a box.... a wooden box filled with paper cards. Libraries cataloged for one reason: to be able to find resources on a shelf. Today, though, we're seeing a growing importance placed on metadata management activities. In an increasingly information-driven world, good metadata is the key ... (Havens and Storey, 2010)

The web is essentially a system of interlinked documents (Berners-Lee et al., 2006). By drawing on library techniques, we can build semantic layers into these documents which can be read by computers and the smart agents described by Berners-Lee. Some computer experts see the Semantic Web as a database of records similar to a national library's union catalogue (Anderson and Rainie, 2010). However, the key to a federation of data is that a new database does not have to be created; actual data remain where they are, rather than being moved to a central location. The key to building semantic layers in a web page or document is to describe them enough to be able to capture their meaning (Mulpeter, 2009). This process is what is known as building an ontology – an unambiguous description of concepts and the relationships between concepts.

A massive project like the Semantic Web requires the application of ontologies, as well as a set of standards or rules, much as we have done for generations in library catalogues. Although library professionals and semantic experts do not typically exchange knowledge, they should be encouraged to do so. Data sharing is a basic tenet of librarianship; libraries of all kinds have been sharing and exchanging cataloguing data and bibliographic records for decades using various library and web standards such as machine-readable cataloguing (MARC) and Z39.50. Organizations such as the Library of Congress (LoC) and the Online Computer Library Center (OCLC) are known for their contributions to data exchange and the development of standards such as those of the Dublin Core Metadata Initiative (DCMI) (Borland, 2007).

Semantic experts in computer science investigate how computers can be programmed to give context to the data we post on websites. However, there seems to be a disconnection between the semantic community on the one hand and librarians on the other, despite the fact that we are both working towards better organization of knowledge. In their research, computer scientists do not seem to realize that semantic control of websites and knowledge objects is a kind of bibliographic control (or cataloguing) writ large, and that many of the principles of access points and language control in librarianship pertain to developing the Semantic Web. Library and Semantic Web professionals should be sharing their knowledge as much as possible, since both groups have a unique view of ontological frameworks and systems of organization.

Health librarians who want to orient themselves to Web 3.0 and the Semantic Web may find that our new cataloguing code, the Resource Description and Access (RDA) standard, is a logical place to start. First, RDA replaced the Anglo-American Cataloguing Rules (AACR2) in 2010 and brings us closer to cataloguing materials for Web 3.0. The DCMI/RDA Task Group is already aware of the importance of interoperable standards and has been converting RDA into the W3C's Resource Description Framework (RDF) – a specification used by semantic practitioners for metadata description. Additionally, the International Federation of Library Associations (IFLA) is translating one of the fundamental guidelines in librarianship, the Functional Requirements for Bibliographic Records (FRBR), into RDF.

To advocate for the development of Web 3.0, the controlled vocabularies we use in our searching should be 'webified' (Hillman, 2007). In fact, members of the DCMI and the RDA Joint Steering Committee have said that libraries should begin to collaborate on updating standards to ensure web compatibility (Hillman et al., 2010). By converting library thesauri and data standards, we ensure a place in the future of the web; however, without conversion into a machine-readable language, none of those services can be integrated. Legacy standards such as the medical subject headings (MeSH) and the National Library of Medicine Classification scheme enjoy respect the world over as organizational tools but are difficult (or impossible) to apply in new digital contexts (Styles et al., 2008).

Web 3.0 is about discovery

Discussion about the web's future is filled with the language of discovery (Anderson and Rainie, 2010). Where Web 2.0 focuses on searching, 'Web 3.0 will be about finding'. Users do not want to search, they want to filter through their networks. Despite our acceptance of all things Google, this hints at the generally poor performance of the current crop of web search engines. Constructing better tools for findability is a central principle of Web 3.0, but this goal should not be at the expense of what we do in libraries. Teaching information and media literacy skills for Web 3.0 will continue to require capable, well informed librarians even if the Semantic Web markedly improves retrieval.

If we want to improve the speed of knowledge transfer in medicine, new ways to cumulate the evidence must be investigated and developed. This work can take place in concert with the Semantic Web, or separately. Consider how much time and energy we invest in grant applications and clinical trial formulation for our users by locating relevant, high-quality studies. This is a burgeoning problem in systematic review searching as well. But since PubMed is no longer the only map of the literature, health librarians must search repeatedly for clinical studies in numerous databases, repositories and websites. To develop better ways of searching the literature, health librarians will need to articulate a vision and idealism comparable to Web 3.0.

One of the goals of the Semantic Web is dealing with information overload or 'information abundance' (Anderson and Rainie, 2010). The root causes of this information problem are easy to identify; as Svenonius says, 'the essential and defining objective of a system for organizing information is to bring *like* information together and to differentiate what is *not* alike' (Svenonius, 2000). However, collocation of information has never been a guiding web principle. It is one of the main reasons Google Scholar is not recommended for literature reviews in medicine, although it excels as a browsing and discovery tool. Google's PageRank has been enormously helpful for searching since 1998 but it does not satisfactorily address the problem of fragmentation. Google recognizes the limitations of its algorithm and has invested in a number of semantic technologies such as Metaweb.com and Rich Snippets (Zaino, 2010). Several other search companies are already in pursuit of their piece of the semantic future.

Web data to 2020

> The semantic web isn't just about putting data on the web. It is about making links, so that a person or machine can explore the web of data. With linked data, when you have some of it, you can find other, related, data. (Berners-Lee et al., 2006)

The DNA of the web is data (Berners-Lee et al., 2001). Typically, health librarians understand the importance of good data and their role in our library catalogues and scientific indexes. But beyond creating metadata, what skills should health librarians bring to managing data in the biosciences (Singer, 2009)? Simply, data curation is the active and ongoing management of data through their life cycle of interest and usefulness to scholarship, science and education (Higgins, 2007). How should we respond to the demands of data curation in medicine, given its importance in scientific investigation? The inability to respond to new demands introduced by the internet is one reason why Silicon Valley and other information professionals have usurped opportunities from librarians. We should not let the same thing happen with scientific data, given their pivotal role, in the future.

According to web experts, the information universe is set to generate billions of new documents by 2020 (Anderson and Rainie, 2010). Knowledge creation in pharmacotherapeutics, genomics and proteomics will also produce data that can be cross indexed (as 'linked data') and foraged to find answers to future health threats and epidemics. Between documents and data, will Google implement a PageRank-like semantic tool to filter this material (Evans, 2008)? The National Library of Medicine has been working on automated indexing projects for more than a decade (Humphrey, 1999) and continues to seek innovative ways to mine the biological data that are created by the National Institutes of Health (NIH). Health librarian-led initiatives are needed to test semantic technologies and to evaluate how to integrate them into our legacy computer systems and organizational practices.

For health librarians, a related organizational challenge in the future will be how to curate repositories of clinical data. Our user groups will want a robust decentralized system that can integrate heterogeneous pre-clinical and clinical data, and the peer-reviewed literature. For clinical trials, researchers already manage multi-site databases and projects through collaborative networking. If health librarians are serious about making biomedical data available on the web, we should think about novel ways to do so through PubMedCentral or a similar international repository.

In 2011, resource description is a necessary part of applying for NIH and Canadian Institutes of Health Research grants. Providing open access to government-funded research is also required in Canada and the USA (Canadian Institutes of Health Research, 2010). In any case, papers published with inadequate metadata in the future will probably remain hidden *in the deep web*. At least one health librarian suggests that standard medical ontologies such as Systematized Nomenclature of Medicine (SNOMED) and the Unified Medical Language System (UMLS) can be used to model and create taxonomies for the Semantic Web (Robu, 2008). Medicine lends itself to semantic mapping and taxonomy development, due to its precise use of language and terminologies.

The Web 3.0 framework

For many decades, the reason why MeSH vocabulary has been effective in searching MEDLINE is its role as a foundational international language in biomedicine. Similarly, web ontology languages such as RDF and the Web Ontology Language (OWL) apply a standard language and aid researchers in retrieving information from the web (Robu, 2008). Other key semantic tools include Friend of a Friend (FOAF), Semantic Protocol and RDF Query Language (SPARQL) and Simple Knowledge Organization System (SKOS) (Legg, 2007; Miles and Pérez-Agüera, 2007). (To gain a general sense of semantic activities in the life sciences, see the W3C Semantic Web Health Care and Life Sciences (HCLS) Interest Group, http://esw.w3.org/HCLSIG.)

In the future, social media may be able to supplement the data generated in our laboratories and clinics, from bench to bedside. Folksonomic tags can be mined from bookmarking sites such as Delicious and Connotea, and potential collaborators and their interests can be found in Facebook and LinkedIn. As an 'index of the crowd', however, tags have limitations (Cho and Giustini, 2008). While tags are acceptable for smaller document collections and citation management, spelling errors, homonym and language confusion multiply as a database scales in size. To account for ambiguities in natural language, some social data will be mappable to various ontologies and frameworks but some human intervention may still be required.

Creating additional semantic-based retrieval techniques that guide consumers to better health information is one goal for the future (Slaughter et al., 2006). Some semantically aware consumers have created their own ontologies (Golbeck and Rothstein, 2008). FOAF is a socio-semantic tool where several million consumers create their own language to describe people, locations, jobs and relationships. FOAF users post and share all kinds of information, photos, and connect their profiles to each other (more 'linked data'), something MySpace and Facebook are only beginning to explore in 2011. Another source of semantic data can be found in social bookmarking and citation management services, where data patterns can be extracted for research papers that are favoured, cited and shared by the public.

Openness has its drawbacks

The openness of the web's data cloud has some drawbacks. For example, information is created faster than internet legislation can be passed to control it. Openness is not an absolute concept and mechanisms will always be needed to prevent criminal use of information. For intellectual works, unless Creative Commons licensing is universally applied to knowledge objects, a strict enforcement of copyright will be increasingly necessary. An example of the tension between open and closed spaces, and copyright's influence in placing barriers before us, is the preview feature in Google Books; there, digital items in the public domain can easily be seen *in toto*, but much content is only available as snippets.

Testing our tolerance and trust of cloud computing are electronic patient record (EPR) systems like Google Health and Microsoft's HealthVault. For some, making EPRs openly accessible and searchable is a threat to privacy. The problem is that every digital act is recorded by multinational corporations, and governments now follow our every move in panopticon-like fashion. Open access to private data is linked to identity theft, and some patient groups have resisted the push to digitize their private health information (Kahn et al., 2010).

Who knew personal information would be this valuable in the digital age? Another problem identified by consumer groups is the repurposing of our personal information by social networking sites without our permission. For example, Facebook allows Google to crawl its pages (Tynan, 2008) and its CEO, Mark Zuckerberg, has said that the 'age of privacy' is over. Extracting personal information is intrusive enough, but particularly so when technology companies use it for other purposes. Health librarians should work closely with legislators to ensure that consumer protections safeguard our personal health information.

Conclusion

In the past decade, web searching has been dominated by 'googling' and iterative searching (Giustini, 2005; Tang and Ng, 2006). Do we really need to search across the whole web for each query? Is that the best solution? Can health librarians devise *greener*, more efficient retrieval methods? As the next logical step, we should find ways to articulate what we want from the web for the next decade.

Social engagement tools are a window to the future of knowledge creation. But should health librarians be showing clinicians how to integrate social media into their research practices? Is this key to organizing and retrieving information in Web 3.0? Health librarians can help their users to build social networking skills and use innovative ways to deliver evidence. This will become even more critical as the web balloons to a trillion documents (Wright, 2009) and the medical literature fragments further.

Today, fewer health professionals are using bricks-and-mortar libraries. The question is, what do we do about it? Does Web 3.0 have the answers? The importance of mobile access to library resources cannot be overstated and, whether it is the Semantic Web or other technology, getting evidence to clinicians means removing barriers to the best filtered content. Our profession must eventually come to terms with how best to make the content in UpToDate and other point-of-care tools openly available.

The Semantic Web is a space of infinite possibility but, like our medical libraries, will be built over time. To realize the Semantic Web, it might be worth reframing the project as an international library initiative. Whatever happens, semantic (or Web 3.0) technology should not adversely affect the 'web experience' for our users, merely augment it (Anderson and Rainie, 2010). What seems clear is that health librarians providing services in the Web 3.0 era will need to adapt constantly as we seek to meet the emerging needs of users.

Note: The list of glossary terms supplied by the authors of this chapter has been incorporated into the full Glossary at the front of the book.

References and further reading

Anderson, J. and Rainie, L. (2010) *The Fate of the Semantic Web*, Pew Research Center Internet and American Life Project, Washington, DC, http://pewinternet.org/Reports/2010/Semantic-Web.aspx.

Atzori, L., Iera, A. and Morabito, G. (2010) The Internet of Things: A survey, *Computer Networks*, **54** (15), 2787-805.

Berners-Lee, T., Hendler, J. and Lassila, O. (2001) The Semantic Web, *Scientific American*, **284** (5), 34–43.

Berners-Lee, T. et al. (2006) A Framework for Web Science, *Foundations and Trends in Web Science*, **1** (1), 1–130.

Borland, J. (2007) A Smarter Web, *Technology Review*, (March/April), www.technologyreview.com/Infotech/18306/.

Canadian Institutes of Health Research (2010) CIHR's Policy on Access to Research Outputs is now in Effect, www.cihr-irsc.gc.ca/e/35683.html.

Carpenter, M. (2002) The Original 73 Rules of the British Museum: a preliminary analysis, *Cataloging and Classification Quarterly*, **35** (1/2), 23–36.

Chepasiuk, R. (1999) Organizing the Internet: the 'core' of the challenge, *American Libraries*, **30** (1), 60–4.

Cho, A. and Giustini, D. (2007) The Semantic Web as a Large, Searchable Catalogue: a librarian's perspective, *The Semantic Universe*, (1 October), http://semanticuniverse.com/articles-semantic-web-large-searchable-catalogue-librarian's-perspective.html.

Cho, A. and Giustini, D. (2008) Web 3.0 and Health Librarians: an introduction, *Journal of the Canadian Health Libraries Association*, **29** (1), 13–18.

Corlain, M. (2009) Web 3.0 or Just 'Augmented Reality + Always Connected / Always in Sync?', *Mihai Corlan*, (September 24), http://corlan.org/2009/09/24/web-3-0-or-just-augmented-reality-always-connected-always-in-sync/.

Evans, W. (2008) Embryonic Web 3.0, *Searcher Magazine*, **16** (1), 12–18.

Fazzinga, B. and Lukasiewicz, T. (2010) Semantic Search on the Web, *Semantic Web – Interoperability, Usability, Applicability (SWJ)*, 1–7, www.kr.tuwien.ac.at/staff/lukasiew/swj10.pdf.

Giustini, D. (2005) How Google is Changing Medicine, *BMJ*, **331**, 1487–8.

Giustini, D. (2007) Web 3.0 and Medicine, *BMJ*, **335**, 1273–4.

Golbeck, J. and Rothstein, M. (2008) Linking Social Networks on the Web with FOAF, *The 17th International World Wide Web Conference Proceedings – WWW 2008, 21–25 April, 2008, Beijing, China*, www.slimtoolbar.com/~golbeck/downloads/foaf.pdf.

Graves, M., Constabaris, A. and Brickley, D. (2007) FOAF: connecting people on the semantic web, *Cataloging and Classification Quarterly*, **43** (3/4), 191–202.

Greenberg, J. and Mendez, E. (2007) Toward a More Library-like Web via Semantic Knitting, *Cataloging and Classification Quarterly*, **43** (3/4), 1–8.

Guha, R., McCool, R. and Miller, E. (2003) Semantic Search. In *Proceedings of the*

Twelfth International World-Wide Web Conference, May, Budapest, Hungary.

Guinard, D. and Trifa, V. (2009) Towards the Web of Things: web mashups for embedded devices. In *Proceedings of WWW (International World Wide Web Conferences), Madrid, Spain, April 2009*, 1–9.

Havens, A. and Storey, T. (2010) The Catalog is Out of the Box, *Next Space: OCLC Newsletter*, (April), www.oclc.org/us/en/nextspace/015/1.htm.

Higgins, S. (2007) Draft DCC Curation Lifecycle Model, *International Journal of Digital Curation*, **2** (2), 82–7.

Hillman, D. (2007) Great Leaps Forward, *Technicalities*, **27** (4), 10–13.

Hillman, D., Coyle, K., Phipps, J. and Dunire, G. (2010) RDA Vocabularies: process, outcome, use, *D-Lib Magazine*, **16** (1/2), http://webdoc.sub.gwdg.de/edoc/aw/d-lib/dlib/january10/hillmann/01hillmann.html.

Humphrey, S. (1999) Automatic Indexing of Documents from Journal Descriptors: a preliminary investigation, *Journal of the American Society of Information Science*, **50** (8), 661–74.

Kahn, J. S., Hilton, J. F., Van Nunnery, T., Leasure, S. and Bryant, K. M. (2010) Personal Health Records in a Public Hospital: experience at the HIV/AIDS clinic at San Francisco General Hospital, *JAMIA: Journal of the American Medical Informatics Association*, **17** (2), 224–8.

Legg, C. (2007) Ontologies on the Semantic Web, *ARIST: Annual Review of Information Science and Technology*, **41**, 432–3.

Lippincott, J. K. (2010) A Mobile Future for Academic Libraries, *Reference Services Review*, **38** (2), 205–13.

Marshall, C. and Shipman, F. (2003) Which Semantic Web? In *Proceedings of the 14th Annual ACM Conference on Hypertext and Hypermedia, 26-30 August 2003, Nottingham*, ACM, 57-66. www.csdl.tamu.edu/~marshall/ht03-sw-4.pdf.

Miles, A. and Pérez-Agüera, J. (2007) SKOS: Simple Knowledge Organisation for the Web, *Cataloging and Classification Quarterly*, **43** (3/4), 69–83.

Mulpeter, D. (2009) The Genesis and Emergence of Web 3.0: a study in the integration of artificial intelligence and the semantic web in knowledge creation, MSc thesis, Dublin Institute of Technology, http://arrow.dit.ie/scschcomdis/23/.

O'Reilly, T. and Battelle, J. (2009) *Web Squared: Web 2.0 five years on*, http://assets.en.oreilly.com/1/event/28/web2009_websquared-whitepaper.pdf.

Robu, I. (2008) Semantic Web Applications in the Biomedical Field, *Journal of the European Association for Health Information and Libraries*, **4** (1), 39–42, www.eahil.net/newsletter/journal_2008_vol4_n1.pdf.

Silva, J. M., Mahfujur Rahman, A. S. M. et al. (2008) Web 3.0: a vision for bridging the gap between real and virtual. In *Proceedings of the 1st ACM International Workshop on Communicability Design and Evaluation in Cultural and Ecological Multimedia Systems, 2008, Vancouver, British Columbia, Canada, 31 October 2008*, ACM, 9–14.

Singer, R. (2009) Linked Library Data Now! *Journal of Electronic Resources Librarianship*, **21** (2), 114–26.

Slaughter, L., Soergel, D. and Rindflesch, T. (2006) Semantic Representation of Consumer Questions and Physician Answers, *International Journal of Medical Information*, **75**, 513–29.

Strickland, M. (2007) The Evolution of Web 3.0. SlideShare presentation, Organic Inc., www.slideshare.net/mstrickland/the-evolution-of-web-30.

Styles, R., Ayers, D. and Shabir, N. (2008) Semantic MARC, MARC 21 and the Semantic Web. In *WWW 2008 Workshop: Linked Data on the Web (LDOW 2008), April 22 2008, Beijing, China*, http://events.linkeddata.org/ldow2008/papers/02-styles-ayers-semantic-marc.pdf.

Svenonius, E. (2000) *The Intellectual Foundation of Information Organization*, MIT Press.

Tang, H. and Ng, J. (2006) Googling for a Diagnosis: use of Google as a diagnostic aid: an internet-based study, *BMJ*, **333**, 1143–5.

Tynan, D. (2008) Five Ways to Defend Your Online Reputation, *PC World*, (23 February), www.pcworld.com/article/id,142721-c,internetnetworking/article.html.

Walsh, A. (2010) QR Codes – using mobile phones to deliver library instruction and help at the point of need, *Journal of Information Literacy*, **4**(1), 55-64, ojs.lboro.ac.uk/ojs/index.php/JIL/article/view/PRA-V4-I1-2010-4.

Wright, A. (2009) Exploring a 'Deep Web' that Google Can't Grasp, *New York Times*, (22 February), www.nytimes.com/2009/02/23/technology/internet/23search.html?th&emc=th.

Zaino, J. (2010) Google, Semantic Web Changing the Content Game, *Internet News: Realtime IT News*, www.internetnews.com/webcontent/article.php/3821231/Google-Semantic-Web-Changing-the-Content-Game.htm.

CHAPTER 15

Conclusion

Paula Younger

Like the printing press, telephone and television before it, the internet has changed forever the way we disseminate and retrieve information.

Both as a group and as individuals, information professionals are rich in imagination, resourcefulness and the ability to innovate, as well as the ability to adopt and adapt to new technology. All of these skills are very apparent from the many and varied examples in this book of how Web 2.0 applications are being used in healthcare information settings.

The sheer variety of the projects outlined here is also testament to the flexibility of Web 2.0 applications, with each service highlighting different features, depending on the needs of their users. Whether it is a practical application to provide information in a more timely and cost-effective manner to users and non-users alike, or a more academic approach, there is a Web 2.0 application that can be used. Some common themes have, however, emerged.

The first of these is the use of the web as a platform. Users are no longer limited to having to use applications on their desktop, laptop or netbook. Online file storage options such as Flickr and Google Docs also mean that users no longer need to rely on memory sticks or external storage. Applications such as haptics and virtual environments such as Second Life offer tremendous potential for the future in all kinds of environments, particularly health.

A second major theme is the trend towards collaborative working. Web applications such as Google Docs, wikis and blogs provide the opportunity for individuals and teams to work on documents and information no matter where they are located. If we assume that, in general, crowds have a higher level of wisdom and knowledge than individuals, then there is also the facility for members of those teams to correct erroneous information. Both information professionals and healthcare professionals are experienced in working collaboratively in multidisciplinary teams to achieve a result: it is now possible to replicate those methods of working in an electronic environment.

A third theme is the use of mobile technology, paving the way for 'web anywhere'. No longer are users tied to a single physical location when it comes to internet access; iPads, wifi hotspots and mobile dongles have made it possible to access the internet from almost anywhere, so long as there is a mobile phone signal.

A fourth theme is the growth of social networking as a method of disseminating information. Facebook has emerged in recent years from being accessible only to Harvard graduates, to become the major social networking site in the world, with over 500 million current users (Facebook, 2010).

A fifth theme is the way in which education delivery has changed. With the advent of virtual worlds and the option to attend lectures and events either in real time or in asynchronous time via podcasts, education is now much more user-focused. This applies whether it is clinical or nursing education for our users, or the option for online continuing professional development (CPD) for ourselves.

A sixth theme is the timeliness of information. Thanks to Twitter, in particular, individuals are now often ahead of the news in their knowledge of what is going on. RSS feeds also enable health professionals to keep up to date with the latest publications in their specialism.

A seventh theme is the lack of need for specialized technical skills. In the early days of the internet, putting a website together required a highly specialized level of technical skills. Now, anyone with a basic level of ICT literacy can quickly create an impressive and interactive website, to be used for all kinds of purposes, from online manuals and textbooks to unsophisticated content management systems where no background programming knowledge is required as the interface facilitates production of web pages and entries. This, combined with the collaborative potential of the internet as we now know it, may be particularly useful in resource-poor settings such as Africa, where the expertise of medical professionals could be harnessed to provide learning and CPD resources that might otherwise be out of reach. In the majority of cases, wikis and blogs in particular require relatively little bandwidth for users to access their basic content.

An eighth theme is flexibility of content. As retweeting and mashups show, content can easily be repurposed to create a result that is more than the sum of its parts. It can be personalized with great ease.

There are many more minor themes that will emerge in the coming months and years, but those listed above are some of the most commonly recurring at present.

This increase in the options for shared working and creativity means that, as information professionals, we must look very carefully at our position as information intermediaries or risk being sidelined. We must be particularly vigilant and vocal about the quality of information, both for ourselves and for our users. We must exercise even more discrimination than when we are dealing with peer-reviewed and anecdotal information.

Those of us who work in environments where any new technology is viewed with suspicion (particularly some government and public sector locations) will need to practise all our resourcefulness, persistence and advocacy skills in encouraging IT departments and board members to support the use of Web 2.0.

We must make sure that we do not lose sight of the importance of dealing ethically with information, particularly where patient information is concerned. Protecting intellectual property and adhering to international copyright law also becomes an important consideration.

We should also beware of relying too heavily on one source alone: in the Web 2.0 world, websites come and go in a very short space of time, so it is always advisable to have at least one back-up information source.

The evolutionary stage of the internet currently termed Web 2.0 offers huge potential benefits in terms of cost-effectiveness, timeliness and personalization in the world of healthcare provision. We are standing at the beginning of a revolution in the way we experience the world: and, as information mediators, we should take every opportunity to reposition ourselves as well qualified information facilitators and educators for our users.

Reference

Facebook (2010) Facebook statistics, www.facebook.com/press/info.php?statistics.

Index